Cyndie Hopewell

Working Effectively With and Within IRBs

A Practical Guide for Investigators, Sponsors, and IRB Members

Working Effectively With and Within IRBs

A Practical Guide for Investigators, Sponsors, and IRB Members

Edited by
Eileen Hilton, MD, and
Deirdre Hall, CCRC, CCRA, CIP

University Publishing Group
Hagerstown, Maryland

University Publishing Group
Hagerstown, Maryland 21740
1(800)654-8188
www.upgbooks.com

Printed in the United States of America
ISBN 1-55572-083-8

Some of the material included in chapter 3 appeared in K. Irvine and E. Hilton, *Ensuring a HIPAA-Compliant Informed Consent Process* (Boston, Mass.: Thomson CenterWatch, 2002).

Contents

Preface

There are numerous excellent resources about institutional review boards—describing what they are, how they work, and why they exist. There are other resources that provide guidance to the IRB administrator, members, and chair. There are few, if any, published works which offer a "how to partner" focus.

We realized the need for a book such as this: a guide to working effectively with IRBs.

For the research sponsors picking up this text: How many times have you been exasperated by an IRB's total rewrite of your informed consent document? Or frustrated by the IRB's seemingly interminable review process?

For the investigators picking up this text: how many times have you had to revise your informed consent form or protocol because of an IRB concern you might not have understood the rationale for?

And finally, for the institutional review "boarders" out there: how many times have you wanted to broadcast your message, "We really aren't trying to delay or prevent research and medical progress"?

An increased understanding of each group's expectations is necessary. We also believe that expectation management should be an important consideration for all clinical research professionals. Further, clinical research professionals would benefit from a direct, practical guide to working together to achieve human subject protections. We believe we offer that here.

We hope you use this text as a vital reference to guide your partnership with IRBs. We need to keep up the good work, but make it better.

—Eileen Hilton and Deirdre Hall
Huntington, Long Island, New York

1

IRB Basics

Eileen Hilton, MD

This chapter is intended to give the reader a historical perspective of human research protections—where it started, how it has progressed, and where it might be heading. Additionally, there is discussion of IRB membership, authority, responsibilities, the Federalwide Assurance (FWA) process, and the sponsor-IRB relationship in the protection of human subjects.

The chapter will focus on:

1.1 A History of Human Subjects Protection
1.2 What an IRB Does
1.3 Responsibilities of IRB Staff
1.4 Federal Regulations, Guidelines, and Institutional Policies
1.5 IRB Registration and the Federalwide Assurance Process
1.6 Take Away Messages

1.1 A HISTORY OF HUMAN SUBJECTS PROTECTION

The Nuremberg Code

The history of human subjects protection dates back to the period after World War II, when the Nuernberg Military Tribunals met in judgment of Nazi wartime activities. The tribunals established 10 principles to be applied during the trials for alleged atrocities committed by Nazi physicians. These became known as *The Nuremberg Code.*[1] The *Code* specified the principles of voluntary consent and the responsibility of researchers to insure that subjects understand the nature of the research to which they are consenting. Subsequently, other groups addressed issues of human subjects protection resulting in *The Declaration of Helsinki* (World Medical Association),[2] the *International Ethical Guidelines for Biomedical Research* (Council for International Organizations of Medical Sciences),[3] and *The Belmont Report* (National Commission for the Protection of Human Subjects of Biomedical and Behavioral Research).[4]

The Declaration of Helsinki

This document, first adopted in 1964, written by physicians for physicians, is considered to be the worldwide standard for medical personnel who conduct human research. It interprets the *Nuremberg* principles and proposes that some risks are acceptable, relative to their importance to humanity as a whole. It has been revised numerous times—most recently in October 2000. The current version questions the ethics of performing placebo-controlled studies when there is alternative treatment available—although it does offer some circumstances when placebo controls would be acceptable, including when there are compelling and scientifically sound reasons for the use of placebo and in investigations into minor conditions when there would not be any additional risk for the recipients.

Comparison of *Nuremberg* and *Helsinki*

Nuremberg was the first research ethics document, whereas *Helsinki* interpreted the ethics principles and matched them with biomedical research reality. *The Nuremberg Code* has never been updated and lacks the flexibility to accommodate changes in clinical research practice. *Helsinki*, on the other hand, has been revised numerous times and may better reflect current trends in human subjects protection. *Helsinki* also opened the door to doing research on potentially vulnerable subjects. For example: *Nuremberg* states that the degree of risk to subjects can never exceed the anticipated benefit of the research to be conducted. *Helsinki* states that some risks are acceptable in relation to the humanitarian importance of the research.

The Belmont Report

The Belmont Report, a result of years of investigations and examinations by the National Commission for the Protection of Human Subjects of Biomedical and Behavioral Research, is critically important, as it serves as one of the major treatises on human subjects research ethics. Although many areas are addressed, *Belmont* is best known for its discussion of three principles as they relate to human subjects protections: (1) respect for persons, (2) beneficence, and (3) justice, including the concept of the equitable selection of subjects.

The following example illustrates the principle of *justice:* A research trial was evaluating an experimental herpes simplex medication and required the participation of both sexual partners—one infected and one uninfected. The protocol was written to include only heterosexual couples. The IRB, applying the principle of justice, questioned whether this exclusion would allow fair sharing of benefits and burdens of the research.

In 1962, the Kefauver-Harris amendments to the Federal Food, Drug, and Cosmetic Act were enacted to more closely regulate the performance of clinical trials involving humans. These amendments delineated requisites that were designed to ensure drug purity and safety, as well as sponsors submission of prior controlled trials. It also resulted in the ability for sponsors to transport experimental drugs across state lines if a prior application to the U.S. Food and Drug Administration (FDA) existed. Similar guidelines were later applied for device trials with the Investigational Device Exemption (IDE).[5] These guidelines depend on a system that includes performance and oversight by the research sponsor, the clinical investigator, and the IRB at the research site.

The Beginnings of the Modern IRB System

In 1966 the U.S. Public Health Service Policy and Procedure Order 129, the forerunner of the modern institutional review board (IRB) system, established the requirement for review of human research by institutional representatives.

The *Code of Federal Regulations* (*CFR*) (the National Research Act), Title 45 Part 46 was proposed by the Department of Health Education and Welfare in 1974.

Subpart A of this *Code*, later referred to as the "Common Rule," is followed by 17 federal agencies. The FDA also established codes that were similar to the U.S. Department of Health and Human Services (DHHS) regulations. 21 *CFR* Parts 50 and 56 are regulations that specifically deal with informed consent and IRBs, respectively.

The International Conference on Harmonisation and its Impact on the IRB System in the U.S.

The International Conference on Harmonisation of Technical Requirements for Registration of Pharmaceuticals for Human Use (ICH) has also addressed issues of human subjects protection. The ICH has and continues to publish guidelines for the performance of clinical research trials.[6] This practical standard permits regulatory authorities in several countries to accept the results of research performed elsewhere and serves to facilitate global research efforts. To date, the FDA does not require compliance with this organization's requirements.

What are the practical effects of this organization and its requirements on sponsors and research sites? IRBs and research sites should familiarize themselves with these standards, as there is a trend toward increased reliance on ICH, especially for international studies; sponsors may request a statement of compliance with ICH guidelines as a condition of approval of a site's participation in a trial.

While ICH has published numerous guidelines, *ICH E6* is a user-friendly guidance tool for good clinical practice (GCP).[7]

Good Clinical Practice AND ICH Guidelines

The purpose of GCP guidelines is to ensure the protection of the safety, rights, and welfare of clinical trial subjects and to insure the quality and integrity of the clinical data that is collected. It boils down to, Have we protected our subjects? and, Is the data collected valid? These comprise the litmus test for conducting quality human subjects research under the principles of GCP.

New Initiatives

In the last few years, as a consequence of the lapses seen in human subjects protection, numerous governmental and nongovernmental organizations and agencies have instituted new initiatives. There are several agencies that have issued or plan to publish reports. Some of the interested parties include the National Human Research Protections Advisory Committee (NHRPAC), the Institute of Medicine's (IOM) Committee on assessing the system for protecting human research subjects, and the Office of Human Research Protections (OHRP) and the FDA.[8] Additionally, in an attempt to maintain some consistency across IRBs, independent accreditation services have emerged, and some organizations plan to have their IRBs accredited by either the Association for the Accreditation of Human Research Protection Programs (AAHRPP) and/or the Partnership for Human Research Protection (PHRP).[9] AAHRPP is a consortium of seven groups, including Public Responsibility in Medicine and Research (PRIM&R), and PHRP is a partnership of two groups—the National Committee for Quality Assurance (NCQA) and the Joint Commission on Accreditation of Healthcare Organizations (JCAHO).

1.2 WHAT AN IRB DOES

IRBs are groups whose foremost duty is to protect the rights and welfare of human subjects. IRB members' familiarity with the investigative site and the local community as well as the investigator's capabilities facilitate considered judgments by an IRB.

IRBs review prospective research protocols and ensure that the design of the planned research affords human subjects the opportunity to give fully informed consent to their voluntary participation in research. In addition, IRB members assess protocols and research plans to evaluate potential risks to subjects, with the goal of protecting them from unreasonable peril. Potential benefits are also assessed that may accrue to the research participant and/or to humanity. The population under study should be assessed. Is it a vulnerable population? Vulnerable populations include children, prisoners, persons who are mentally disabled, pregnant women, fetuses, and the economically or educationally disadvantaged. In addition, members of other groups, including students and employees, may be considered vulnerable.

To summarize, properly functioning IRBs protect subjects by ensuring unbiased selection of subjects, ensuring subjects' full and non-coerced informed consent, assessing risks to subjects, and protecting privacy.

Medical Device Trials and IRBs

In medical device studies, IRBs must ascertain whether devices pose a "significant risk," or a "nonsignificant risk." If IRBs consider a device to be a "significant risk," the sponsor must submit a full investigational device exemption (IDE) application to the FDA for approval. The FDA, in its information sheets, describes criteria that are helpful to a determination of significant versus nonsignificant risk. Examples of devices that pose significant risk are products that are intended as implants and that present a potential for serious risk, or products that are intended for use in supporting or sustaining life and in diagnosing, curing, or treating disease.[10] Please note that the determination of significant risk in device trials should not be confused with, and is not analogous to, a determination of "minimal risk" in other research that may be presented to the IRB. The determination of which protocols present *minimal risk* is discussed further in chapter 2.

After a trial begins, IRBs must conduct meaningful continuing review to ensure that subjects are protected from unforeseen risks. IRBs must be notified of any unanticipated problems that pose risks to subjects or others, including physical or psychological injury to subjects, improper disclosure of private information, economic loss, or other potentially harmful occurrences.

What Constitutes an IRB?

An IRB must have a minimum of five voting members. Membership requirements include one scientist and one nonscientific constituent. Additionally, membership should include an individual who has no known affiliation with the organization conducting the research. This unaffiliated member may be recruited from the community. Groups that may contain appropriate individuals for this role include the clergy, educators, businesspersons, and homemakers. This individual should be familiar with the community and any special issues that may apply to the population of potential research subjects. Unquestionably, the ethnic composition of the community should be considered in this choice, as it should in the selection of other potential members of the IRB.

This community member should be independent of any interests held by the institution and should not be subject to undue influence or coercion from any quarter. As the same person may also serve as the nonscientific member, but note that it is a requirement that a "lay" or nonscientific member be present at every meeting, as the community member may not always be available to attend meetings. It is probably prudent to have two separate individuals serve these different functions. Many IRBs include lawyers, as IRBs must be able to interpret federal and state requirements and guidance.

The general membership should also reflect the gender and ethnic composition of the community it serves. Individuals of different gender or ethnic background may view a protocol very differently. Such diversity is important in ensuring comprehensive review. A lack of diversity in IRB membership has recently been the focus of criticism by OHRP and others.

What Types of Individuals Should Be on an IRB?

Representatives from more than one profession should be included on IRBs. As IRBs review protocols from a number of scientific specialties, appropriately knowledgeable reviewers or consultants should be available. Although it is not an explicit requirement, it is advisable to have a specialist review or be present during deliberations: for example, a pediatrician for pediatric protocols or psychiatrist for psychiatric trials. Consultants may be very useful if your IRB membership lacks expertise in a particular discipline.

How Can Deficiencies in IRB Membership Impact Sponsors?

If an IRB is inspected by regulatory agencies and is found to have a lack of diversity or expertise, research could be suspended, resulting in delays or negative consequences for all involved. Sponsor representatives, as part of routine site qualification, should check the roster of the IRB and ensure that it meets federal assurance standards. These rosters may be checked during routine and for-cause audits and or inspections.[11] In the past, IRB staff reported to administrators within the grants or clinical trials offices of their organization. This may be imprudent, as conflict of interest issues are a concern when the administrative staff is linked to the research business generation arm of the institution.

1.3 RESPONSIBILITIES OF IRB STAFF

There are two general categories of staff: the IRB chair and administrative staff. Their roles are discussed more comprehensively in chapter 8.

IRB Chair

- Performs oversight of all of the activities of the IRB, including leadership of the IRB.
- Maintains current knowledge of ethical issues, institutional policies, and federal, state, and local regulations, and oversees compliance with all.
- Establishes organizational policies.
- Confirms compliance with federal assurances.
- Represents the organization in discussions with federal and state authorities.
- Works with staff and investigators to ensure that human subjects are protected.
- Oversees IRB staff.
- Maintains programs to train IRB staff, committee members, and individuals who are involved in research at the organization.
- Selects investigators for audits and ensures performance and documentation of the audit process.

IRB Administrative Staff

- Responsible for helping to protect human subjects.

- Assist the chair in performing the responsibilities outlined above.
- Assist in maintaining compliance with federal and organizational policies.
- Ensure compliance with federal assurances.
- Assist in training research professionals and the IRB staff.
- Monitor compliance with organizational and federal regulations.

What Are the Implications for the Sponsor and Investigational Team?

Customarily, IRB administrative staff will be investigators' first point of contact. Competent IRB administrative staff can assist investigators in obtaining the information and assistance they require to effectively conduct research with human subjects. When IRB staff members cannot provide the assistance needed, they will contact the chairperson of the IRB for assistance.

1.4 FEDERAL REGULATIONS, GUIDELINES, AND INSTITUTIONAL POLICIES

The regulations that dictate the performance of human research include 21 *CFR* 50 and 56 and 45 *CFR* 46. Regulations under Title 21 pertain to food and drugs, and research conducted under the jurisdiction of the Food and Drug Administration, Title 45, pertains to public welfare and research conducted under the jurisdiction of the DHHS.

The initial review and ongoing surveillance of the trial are carried out in compliance with the regulatory oversight of one or both of these agencies—the Office for Human Research Protections (OHRP), on behalf of the DHHS, and/or the FDA for products regulated by this agency. When research involving products regulated by the FDA is funded, supported, or conducted by FDA and/or DHHS, both the DHHS and FDA regulations apply. Since there are differences in the regulations between these two agencies, the IRB may need to determine under which jurisdiction a research project falls.

IRB Authority

An IRB serves to protect human subjects in its affiliated institution(s). It has the authority to approve, require modification in, or reject initial research proposals, as well as to suspend or terminate ongoing research. If an IRB suspends or terminates research, the investigator, institutional officials, and governmental authorities must receive notification of these actions. An IRB also has the authority to monitor and audit research at the institution.

How Often Is this Power Exercised?

In a 1998 report by the National Institutes of Health (NIH) that evaluated the IRB system, only 37 percent of the chairs queried reported that they had used their authority to suspend or terminate approval of one or more research studies.[12] The federal government has given its agencies (the FDA and OHRP) the authority to enforce the statutes and regulations that guide human research. These agencies are charged with the oversight of IRBs and have the power to suspend or terminate research either individually or organization-wide, at their discretion.

How Aggressive Is this Oversight?

Organizational Implications

Governmental regulatory groups are inspecting IRBs more frequently. If an inspection of a clinical site or an IRB shows serious compliance issues, the FDA and OHRP may suspend or terminate the clinical investigation. Sites and sponsors should be aware that results of inspections from one agency may be shared with the other and trigger an additional inspection. The FDA may also disqualify or suspend a clinical investigator if there has been repeated or deliberate failure to comply with applicable regulatory requirements, or the clinical investigator has submitted false information to the sponsor, or, if applicable, to the FDA. A disqualified clinical investigator cannot receive investigational drugs, biologics, or devices. The FDA publishes the names of clinical investigators who have been disqualified or "totally restricted." There is a difference between "totally restricted" (absent reinstatement) and "restricted" investigators. The latter may still receive investigational products, provided they conduct regulated studies in accordance with the restrictions specified in their agreement with FDA and all applicable regulatory requirements. The FDA also maintains lists for restricted clinical investigators at its website (see "Useful Websites" at the end of this book).[13]

In certain circumstances, the government may decide to litigate. Although this is unusual, criminal provisions of the Food and Drug Act can be applied to clinical investigators and IRB members.

Implications for Sponsors

The FDA can reject product submissions and can withdraw approvals previously granted if new information regarding the integrity of the data or study conduct is brought to light. The Application Integrity Policy also can be implemented when there are issues surrounding the data quality and integrity. If this policy is applied, FDA may suspend the review of all applications until the problem has been resolved.[14] Further discussion of these issues can be found in chapters 6 and 7.

Do IRBs Really Protect Subjects?

Protection of research subjects depends on IRBs to ensure compliance with regulations that serve to protect human subjects. After several instances of inadequate protection of human subjects, federal agencies were concerned about the ability of our system to safeguard research subjects.

In 1998, a report by the Office of the Inspector General (OIG), "Protecting Human Research Subjects," warned that the effectiveness of IRBs was in jeopardy.[15] In another report, when IRB chairs, members, and investigators were asked if their IRB protects human subjects, the responses indicated that only 18 percent of the chairs, 21 percent of the members, and 30 percent of the investigators thought IRBs did protect subjects.[16] Numerous suggestions were made in an attempt to improve the quality of human subjects protection.

One of the most important issues that was addressed dealt with the process of continuing review. A consistent finding of the OIG was the minimal time spent by IRBs on continuing review, with comments such as "hurried" or "superficial." They also noted that these reviews were limited to paperwork submitted by researchers, and that there was a lack of on-site monitoring. The report cited heightened workload pressures, limited feedback on multi-site trials, inadequate feedback on FDA actions against investigators, a shortage of members with scientific expertise, and minimal outside representation.[17]

In April 2000, a follow-up report was issued describing, among other things, actions taken after the first report. In the time interval between the two filings, on-site investigations had been conducted at 10 institutions by OHRP (then OPRR—the Office for Protection from Research Risks). Similarly, the FDA had markedly increased its number of on-site investigations (213 in 1997, 253 in 1998, and 336 in 1999).[18] OHRP's reviews resulted in the suspension of research at seven institutions. But, despite this evidence of increasingly stringent oversight, the April 2000 report remained critical of the state of human subjects protection provided by the IRB system.

Specifically, the April 2000 report cited a lack of progress in (1) changing federal IRB requirements to make them more flexible but accountable for the protection of human subjects, (2) enhancing protection for subjects beyond the initial review, (3) requiring stronger educational programs for investigators and IRB members, (4) increasing oversight by institutions and IRBs regarding conflict of interest issues, (5) moderating workload pressures of IRBs, and (6) improving the federal oversight process. One impediment described by the report was difficulty in effecting changes to the "Common Rule" (the core policy on human subjects protection, enacted in 1991, referenced earlier). A significant hindrance to reform was the need for consensus among the 17 federal agencies that must approve any changes to the "Common Rule." On a more promising note, the authors of the report cited some improvements, for example, that NIH and FDA required the sharing of information collected by data safety monitoring boards (DSMBs).[19] Information regarding investigator misconduct was also being shared between agencies, and agencies have begun educational initiatives.

Problems for Investigative Sites—Changing Expectations of Oversight Agencies

It has become increasingly difficult to determine what is expected and how to meet the expectations of regulatory officials. The situation would be more manageable if the written regulations were the only ones institutional officials and IRBs had to be concerned about. The protection of human subjects continues to evolve, and oversight agencies may implement "requirements" before they are formally endorsed as regulations. Many clinical research professionals use information regarding past disciplinary actions at other organizations as their source of the latest information and to predict what might be expected of them by federal inspectors.

The "Common Rule," which is followed by 17 federal agencies, may not be adaptable enough to deal with new scientific developments and ethical issues. Different agencies may have different interpretations of the rule, which can cause inconsistencies in its oversight and enforcement. This dilemma is becoming increasingly frustrating for institutions and IRBs, who want to comply with regulations but are unsure of what additional guidance they should follow.

How Have the Agencies Responded?

As a result of reports that called for a more unified approach to the oversight of human research, the OPRR has moved to the DHHS and was renamed the Office of Human Research Protections (OHRP). The move was deemed necessary to broaden the scope of the office and initiate reforms for all of the governmental agencies subscribing to the "Common Rule." There are several differences between the original agency and its successor. First, OHRP oversees only human research. Second, OHRP's responsibilities are more comprehensive, including leadership for all agencies that conduct or fund research under the "Common Rule." The FDA is included as one of these agencies, but still maintains its specific oversight and regulatory responsibilities.[20] In addition to OHRP, a National Human Research Protections Advisory Committee (NHRPAC) was formed.

The FDA also established the Office for Good Clinical Practice (OGCP) within the Office of the Commissioner and its Office of Science Coordination and Communication. This organization's role is to improve the "conduct and oversight of clinical research and to ensure the protection of participants in FDA-regulated clinical research."[21] The new FDA agency is expected to help ensure consistency of human subjects protections implementation. It is also expected that the OHRP and OGCP will work together toward this common goal.

On the Horizon?

It has been proposed that yet another agency is to be formed—a single federal oversight group that would be named the National Office of Human Research Protection Oversight (NOHPRO). This proposal has been met with varying degrees of enthusiasm. Critics have claimed that it "will lead to confusion of hegemony and administrative responsibility with respect to implementation of federal regulations."[22]

Do IRBs Really Protect Human Subjects?

If an IRB performs its required functions, it helps ensure the protection of human subjects. However, it is inappropriate to rely solely on an IRB to do this job. Investigators, sponsors, and institutional officials equally share the responsibility for human subjects protection. It is evident from recent events that there is room for added improvement in the realm of human subjects protections.

1.5 IRB REGISTRATION AND THE FWA PROCESS

IRB registration and FWA are two separate issues. The following information is found on the OHRP website, *http://OHRP.osophs.dhss.gov.*

Should an IRB Be Registered?

Registration is required for all IRBs designated under an OHRP FWA. For others, it is voluntary and not currently required by the FDA. Although it is not required, any IRB that desires to register may do so with DHHS/OHRP. A unique number will be assigned to the newly registered IRB.

Should an IRB File an FWA?

This discussion will focus on the current system for assurance—FWA. Please note that the assurance system was simplified in 2000. Section 103(a) of the federal policy (the "Common Rule") for the protection of human subjects requires that each institution "engaged" in federally supported human subject research file an "assurance" of protection for human subjects. This assurance serves to formalize the commitment to protect human subjects.[23] If an institution is collaborating with other sites doing research, the primary site must ensure that all collaborators engaged in the research hold an assurance prior to their initiation of the research.[24]

Who May File an FWA and Can an Organization Rely on Another Organization's IRB?

Any registered institution may file an FWA with DHHS/OHRP. An organization requires its own FWA, but can rely on another organization's IRB if the arrangement is agreeable to both parties and satisfies the guidelines for knowledge of the local research context. This is regardless of the IRB's geographic location relative to the institution and the research.

How Can an Off-Site IRB Be Cognizant of Another Area's Research Context?

A member or members of the reviewing IRB may be familiar with the local research environment. Additionally, members or consultants affiliated with the collaborating organization may participate in the review process (physical attendance or through video-teleconference or teleconference) at meetings of the IRB. If they are unable to attend in person, a satisfactory written evaluation may be submitted and the committee may waive the attendance requirement.

Even if institutions elect to rely upon another organization's IRB, it remains the responsibility of the organization where the research is taking place to maintain an institutional system to protect human subjects.[25] Any responsibilities delegated to the IRB of record should be put in writing. An institution that requests another IRB to review for it is still responsible for the protection of human subjects that is ongoing at its site, educating its research community, and implementing oversight to ensure compliance with the determinations of the reviewing IRB. This is discussed in more detail in chapter 8, part E, "Legal Counsel for Human Subjects Protection Programs."

When an institution has a local IRB, the institution is required to provide administrative support, space, and facilities, and to designate an institutional official to oversee the IRB's functions.

What about Investigators Who Do Not Have a Local IRB? How Does This System Affect Them?

When investigators conduct federally supported research, they are subject to all of the usual human protections requirements, and therefore must enter into an arrangement with an institution that has filed an FWA. This can be done by using a template supplied by the OHRP, the "Unaffiliated Investigator Agreement" available on its website.[26] The agreement is with the institution with an FWA and need not be forwarded to OHRP. Additionally, a group of private practitioners may file an FWA for its practice group.

Are There Any Other Requirements for Institutions Under the FWA System?

There are educational requirements as follows: the OHRP regulation states that the institutional signatory official, the human protections administrator, and the IRB chairperson must complete the OHRP basic educational modules (or equivalent to the OHRP modules) prior to submitting the assurance. Also, IRB members and staff must complete appropriate training before reviewing human subject research. Many IRBs additionally require that investigators complete human subjects protections training. This is a requirement for participation in NIH-funded clinical research.[27]

Does this Assurance Cover Non-Federally Funded Research?

Yes, federal assurances may cover non-federally funded research if the IRB chooses to configure its assurance in this manner. Most do. However, IRBs can elect to separate oversight by the source of the research funding.

What about Other Accreditation Groups?

There are independent accreditation agencies that have begun to evaluate IRBs. As previously mentioned, the major players in this area are AAHRPP and PHRP. The process of accreditation is very labor intensive and expensive, but many IRBs are considering applying for accreditation by one or both of these agencies.

Implications of the FWA for Sponsors

When a research site is being qualified, there is an increased level of comfort when an organization holds an FWA or is accredited by an independent agency. Either of these suggests that the membership roster has withstood outside review and that ongoing research meets minimum standards. IRBs that provide an assurance statement in lieu of a membership roster should document the assurance number and the assurance's expiration date.

The Relationship between the IRB and the Research Sponsor

It is sometimes perceived that IRBs delay or impede human subjects research. When sponsors, IRBs, and investigators are partners in the research process, delays are minimized for those attempting to gain approval for new agents or devices.

1.6 TAKE AWAY MESSAGES

- Although there is still room for improvement, human subjects protection have made great strides in the last 50 years.
- Regulation and guidance have evolved over the years including *Nuremberg, Helsinki, Belmont,* and the ICH guidelines.
- Be familiar with the ICH guidelines—these are an international standard for good clinical practice. FDA does not yet require compliance with this organization's requirements, but the guidelines have been published in the *Federal Register.*
- Best GCP resource—*ICH E6.*
- GCP litmus test: Have human subjects been protected and is the data collected valid?
- Federal agencies with authority in human subjects protections include the FDA and the OHRP (from the DHHS).
- Good resources to keep current are listed in Appendix B, "Useful Websites."
- Regulation is not a substitute for ethical conduct.
- A properly functioning IRB protects study subjects by ensuring unbiased selection, full and non-coercive informed consent, assessment of risk, and protection of privacy.
- IRBs should have a minimum of five members, including one scientist, one nonscientist, and one nonaffiliated member. Lawyers are often useful members, and can serve as the community member if they are not affiliated with the institution.
- IRB membership should be diverse in gender and ethnicity and should reflect the community the IRB serves.
- When is it appropriate to contact an IRB? Any question concerning subjects' safety or data integrity.
- The IRB has the authority to approve, require modification in, or reject initial research proposals, as well as to suspend or terminate ongoing research.
- Institutions should register their IRBs and consider filing an FWA that serves to formalize the commitment to protect human subjects. Accreditation by an outside organization should be considered as well.
- When sponsors, IRBs, and investigators partner in the research process, delays are minimized for those attempting to gain approval for new agents or devices.

NOTES

1. *The Nuremberg Code,* "Permissible Medical Experiments," *Trials of War Criminals before the Nuernberg Military Tribunals under Control Council Law No. 10: Nuernberg, October 1946 - April 1949* (Washington, D.C.: U.S. Government Printing Office, n.d., vol. 2): 181-2; *http://ohsrod.nih.gov/nuremberg.php3,* accessed 10 July 2002.

2. World Medical Association, *The Declaration of Helsinki, http://www.wma.net/e/ethicsunit/helsinki.htm,* accessed 10 July 2004.

3. CIOMS and WHO, *International Ethical Guidelines for Biological Research Involving Human Subjects* (Geneva: CIOMS, 1993), *www.cioms. ch.*

4. U.S. Department of Health, Education and Welfare, *The Belmont Report* (Washington, D.C.: U.S. Government Printing Office, 1988, 201/778-80319 GPO 887-809); originally published in 44 *Federal Register* (18 April 1979), 23192-7; *http://ohrp. osophs.dhhs.gov/human subjects/guidance/belmont.htm,* accessed 10 July 2002.

5. *The Evolution of US Drug Law, www.fda.gov/fdac/special/newdrug/benlaw.html,* accessed 10 July 2002.

6. The International Conference on Harmonisation, *http://www.ich.org/*, accessed 10 July 2002.

7. ICH GCP Guidelines—E6, *http://www.ifpma.org/pdf>ifpma/e6.pdf,* accessed 28 May 2002.

8. National Human Research Protections Advisory Committee, *ohrp.osophs. dhhs.gov/nhrpac/nhrpac.htm,* accessed 10 July 2002.

9. PRIM&R, *What is AAHRP? http://www.primr.org/aahrpp.html,* accessed 10 July 2002.

10. FDA Information Sheets: *Guidance for Institutional Review Boards and Clinical Investigators* 1998 Update, *http://www.fda.gov/oc/ohrt/irbs/devices.html,* accessed 10 July 2002.

11. Ibid.

12. DHHS, *Report of the Office of Inspector General; Institutional Review Boards—A Time for Reform, http://oig.hhs.gov/oei/reports/a276.pdf,* accessed 10 July 2002.

13. FDA, Office of Regulatory Affairs, *Compliance References: Bioresearch Monitoring, http://www.fda.gov/ora/compliance_ ref/bimo/dis_res_assur.htm,* accessed 20 April 2002.

14. FDA, Office of Regulatory Affairs, *Compliance Issues: Application Integrity Policy, http://www.fda.gov/ora/compliance _ref/aip_page.html,* accessed 21 June 2002.

15. *OEI-01-97-00197* (Washington, D.C.: DHHS, 2000).

16. NIH, Office of Extramural Research 1998, *http://ohrp.osophs. dhhs.gov/hsp_report/hsp_final_rpt.pdf,* accessed 21 June 2002.

17. Ibid.

18. DHHS, Report of the Office of Inspector General, *Protecting Human Research Subjects: Status of Recommendations (OEI-01-97-00197: 4/00), http://oig.hhs.gov/oei/reports/oei-01-97-00197.pdf,* accessed 21 June 2002.

19. Ibid.

20. Statement of Greg Koski, Director OHRP, 28 September 2000, *http://ohrp.osophs.dhhs.gov/references/tkoski.htm,* accessed 10 May 2002.

21. Establishment of the Office for Good Clinical Practice, 26 October 2001, FDA, *http://www.fda.gov/oc/gcp/ogcp.html,* accessed 20 May 2002.

22. Eric M. Meslin, "Comment Letter on Ethical and Policy Issues in Research Involving Human Participants," 26 January 2001, *http://www.aamc.org/research/dbr/compliance/nbaccommentletter.htm,* accessed 10 May 2002.

23. OHRP, "IRB Registration and Assurance Filing Procedures," *ohrp.osophs. dhhs.gov/humansubjects/assurance/refinfo.htm,* accessed 10 May 2002.

24. Ibid.

25. See item (c) of OHRP guidance, "Knowledge of Local Research Context," 21 July 2000, *http://ohrp.osophs.dhhs.gov/humansubjects/guidance/local.htm,* accessed 10 June 2002.

26. Federalwide Assurance, OHRP, *http://ohrp.osophs.dhhs.gov/human subjects/assurance/unaflsup.rtf,* accessed 10 May 2002.

27. *http://ohrp.osophs.dhhs.gov/humansubjects/assurance/unaflsup.rtf.*

2

The IRB Review Process

Deirdre Hall, CCRC, CCRA, CIP

This chapter will focus on issues and procedures that are relevant to the IRB review process. The mechanisms of IRB review (that is, full board review versus expedited review) and the types of IRB review (that is, initial review, adverse events, amendments, and continuing review) will also be discussed.

The chapter will address these areas:

2.1 Criteria for IRB Approval
2.2 Relationship between Sponsor, Investigator, and IRB Review
2.3 What Happens to a Proposal When It Is Submitted to an IRB?
2.4 Planning Genetic Research that Is "IRB Approvable"
2.5 Common Reasons for IRB Deferral, Rejection, or Delay
2.6 Suggestions for Avoiding Delays in the Review Process—Improving Efficiency without Sacrificing Quality or Integrity
2.7 The IRB Wants to Change the Protocol—Implications for Multi-Center Trials
2.8 Effectively and Tactfully Managing What Looks Like IRB "Nitpicking"
2.9 How Can Sponsors and Investigators Navigate the IRB Review Process?
2.10 What Can the IRB Do to Facilitate Review?
2.11 Take Away Messages

2.1 CRITERIA FOR IRB APPROVAL

To the untrained, IRB regulations may seem to be fairly straightforward. Deeper consideration will show, however, that the functions of IRBs are complex, and their role extraordinarily integral to the protection of human subjects. Fortunately, there is a well-defined list of requirements that must be met before an IRB can approve a research project.

The requirements for IRB approval are grounded in the basic ethical principles of the National Commission's 1979 *The Belmont Report for the Protection of Human Subjects of Biomedical and Behavioral Research*—often referred to as *The Belmont Report* or simply *Belmont.*[1] These principles include *respect for persons, beneficence,* and *justice.*

The *Belmont* Principles and the *Code of Federal Regulations*

Consistent with the principle of *respect for persons*, it is required that informed consent be sought from each prospective subject or the subject's legally authorized representative and that this process will be documented (unless specifically waived by the IRB.)[2] Additionally, when appropriate, the research plan must make adequate provision for monitoring collected data to ensure the safety of subjects, protect their privacy, and maintain the confidentiality of data.[3]

Consistent with the principle of *beneficence*, the regulations require that risks to subjects be minimized by using procedures that are consistent with sound research design and that do not expose subjects to any unnecessary risk.[4] Whenever appropriate, researchers should use procedures that would ordinarily be performed on the subjects for diagnostic or treatment purposes. This is a practical interpretation of the themes "do no harm" and "maximize possible benefits and minimize possible harms." Clinical intervention protocols, for example, should be written with consideration and application of accepted standards of care for the disease or condition under investigation.

The next requirement may present a challenge for an IRB:

> Risks to subjects should also be reasonable in relation to anticipated benefits, if any, to subjects and the importance of the knowledge that may be expected to result. In evaluating risks and benefits, the IRB should consider only those risks and benefits that may result from the research as distinguished from the risks and benefits the subjects would receive in standard care. The IRB should not consider possible long-range effects of applying knowledge gained in the research as among those research risks that fall within the purview of its responsibility.[5]

Finally, consistent with the ethical principle of *justice*, selection of subjects must be equitable.[6] In making an assessment that selection is equitable, an IRB should evaluate the purpose of the research and the setting in which the study will be conducted. An IRB should be particularly cognizant of the special problems of research that involve vulnerable populations, such as children, prisoners, pregnant women, fetuses, students and employees, mentally disabled persons, and economically or educationally disadvantaged persons. This is a complicated assessment that can be broken down into three components: (1) purposes of the research, (2) setting in which the research will be conducted, and (3) special populations.

The purpose of the research must be defined (usually described as specific objectives) in the body of the protocol. It is difficult for an IRB to approve a protocol in which there is a lack of clearly defined objectives. Historical cases of human experimentation (for example, medical war crimes in Nazi concentration camps) did not meet this basic requirement. In these "studies," the research design was undefined and appeared to be indiscriminate.

Industry sponsors are usually skilled at defining objectives, but some investigators who design their own research may have more difficulty with this. An increasing number of industry sponsors conduct "fishing expeditions,"—that is, projects designed to collect tissue samples that go exploring without any defined objective. This is because the sponsors are not yet sure what they hope to find. Several strategies that investigators can use to assure that their genetic testing or other tissue collection protocols will pass an IRB's "sniff test" are described later in this chapter.

The research setting may be used to refer to various aspects of research, including, but not limited to, the location(s) where subjects will be seen and the conditions under which their consent will be sought.

Finally, under the approvability requirements,[7] reference to *special populations* is especially important. The principle of *justice*, as defined in *The Belmont Report*, in part incorporates the theme that "equals ought to be treated equally." Extra protections for potentially vulnerable or "unequal" groups are included in the "Common Rule" (45 *CFR* 46). The U.S. Food and Drug Administration (FDA) has adopted most of the provisions to protect children that are outlined in the "Common Rule." Regardless of what is written in the *Code of Federal Regulations*, IRBs and researchers are ethically obligated to satisfy the requirements of the principle of justice.

2.2 RELATIONSHIP BETWEEN SPONSOR, INVESTIGATOR, AND IRB REVIEW

While informed consent will be addressed in much greater detail in chapter 3, "Consent Issues," it will also be discussed here as it relates to IRB review. The vast majority of industry sponsors prepare an informed consent template for investigational sites. This text refers repeatedly to the idea of partnerships between IRBs, investigators, and sponsors. Such partnerships should include associates who assist each other in the protection of human subjects. A functioning partnership should result in a system of checks and balances. If the sponsor fails to include an important element in the informed consent, a check by the investigator may catch the lapse. Similarly, if the investigator errs, it is hoped that the IRB will detect errors or omissions.

Some investigators spend little or no time considering the template: whether it meets the local and federal IRB requirements or whether it adequately reflects the protocol. It may appear that IRBs spend a disproportionate amount of time reviewing the consent document, relative to the amount of time spent reviewing the protocol or other research activities. Best practice calls for review by all stakeholders. It is now common practice for investigators to send modifications to the sponsor-provided consent form to the sponsor for pre-approval before it is submitted to an IRB. Why is this done? A sponsor may have legal issues with some of the changed language. Or a sponsor may feel that it is improving the consent document. Whatever the case, these matters should be turned around efficiently, lest significant delays result in the trial being "bumped" from the IRB's agenda.

Similarly, after an IRB suggests consent form changes, sponsors may ask to see the changes and take issue with some of them. If an IRB does not agree with the sponsor's language, the "approved" consent document will not be altered. The IRB has the final word. The sponsor can then decide whether or not the trial will proceed at that site. To decrease delays in final approval, the sponsor may choose to limit its comments and changes to substantive issues.

2.3 WHAT HAPPENS TO A PROPOSAL WHEN IT IS SUBMITTED TO AN IRB?

When an investigator submits a protocol to an IRB, a number of steps typically follow. An IRB always establishes and publishes defined submission deadlines. The purpose is to allow time for the IRB staff to accomplish several things prior to the full board meeting. For busy IRBs, organizing an IRB meeting agenda is a time-consuming undertaking.

IRBs have a defined application or submission form that must be reviewed in advance of a convened meeting. The IRB staff should evaluate submissions regarding possible conflicts of interest for the investigator (financial or otherwise), and to evaluate methods to protect subjects, monitor safety, ensure collection of informed consent, and identify subjects equitably. The IRB staff should ensure that the proposed investigator has not been disqualified or restricted by the FDA. In addition, the consent form should be reviewed to ensure that the essential elements are present. These activities are time-consuming.

For both sponsors and investigators, *respect for IRB submission deadlines* is essential to a successful working relationship with the IRB. Late submissions accompanied by pleas for exceptions are the bane of all IRB staff members.

Types of IRB Review

There are two types of IRB review: *full review* and *expedited review*.[8] The primary difference between full review and expedited review is that full review must take place at a convened meeting of the committee, whereas an expedited review can be conducted by an individual designated by an IRB.

How does an IRB decide whether an item qualifies for expedited review?

The IRB administrator must consider the proposed activity and determine whether it meets requisite criteria. The most common use of the expedited review process is the review of minor changes in previously approved research. Other research activities may qualify for expedited review if they fall within a category on the DHHS/FDA November 1998 "Expedited Review List."[9] The categories apply only to research activities that present no more than minimal risk to subjects. Since there is frequently confusion about what qualifies under these categories, it is useful to review them here.

What are the categories that allow expedited review?

The summarized categories of research that may be reviewed by an IRB through an expedited procedure are as follows:

1. Clinical studies of drugs and medical devices only when condition (a) or (b) is met. Condition (a): Research on drugs for which an investigational new drug application (21 *CFR* Part 312) is not required. Condition (b): Research on medical devices for which (i) an investigational device exemption application (21 *CFR* Part 812) is not required; or (ii) the medical device is cleared/approved for marketing and the medical device is being used in accordance with its cleared/approved labeling.
2. Collection of blood samples by finger stick, heel stick, ear stick, or venipuncture as follows: (a) from healthy, nonpregnant adults who weigh at least 110 pounds. For these subjects, amounts drawn may not exceed 550 ml in an eight-week period and collection may not occur more frequently than two times per week; or (b) from other adults and children, considering the age, weight, and health of the subjects, the collection procedure, the amount of blood to be collected, and the frequency with which it will be collected. For these subjects, the amount drawn may not exceed the lesser of 50 ml or 3 ml per kg in an eight-week period, and collection may not occur more frequently than two times per week.
3. Prospective collection of biological specimens for research purposes by noninvasive means.
4. Collection of data through noninvasive procedures (not involving general anesthesia or sedation) routinely employed in clinical practice, excluding procedures involving x-rays or microwaves.

When medical devices are employed, they must be cleared/approved for marketing.

5. Research involving materials (data, documents, records, or specimens) that have been collected or will be collected solely for nonresearch purposes (such as medical treatment or diagnosis). Some research in this category may be exempt from the DHHS regulations for the protection of human subjects (45 *CFR* 46).
6. Collection of data from voice, video, digital, or image recordings made for research purposes.
7. Research on individual or group characteristics or behavior (including, but not limited to, research on perception, cognition, motivation, identity, language, communication, cultural beliefs or practices, and social behavior) or research employing surveys, interviews, oral history, focus group, program evaluation, human factors evaluation, or quality assurance methodologies. Some research in this category may also be exempt from the DHHS regulations for the protection of human subjects.
8. Continuing review of research previously approved by the convened IRB as follows: (a) where (i) the research is permanently closed to enrollment of new subjects; (ii) all subjects have completed all research-related interventions; and (iii) the research remains active only for long-term follow up of subjects; or (b) when no subjects have been enrolled and no additional risks have been identified; or (c) when the remaining research activities are limited to data analysis.
9. Continuing review of research that is not conducted under an investigational new drug application or investigational device exemption, when categories (2) through (8) do not apply, but the IRB has determined and documented at a convened meeting that the research involves no greater than minimal risk and no additional risks have been identified.

What Is Minimal Risk?

Minimal risk means that the "probability and magnitude of harm or discomfort anticipated in the research are not greater, in and of themselves, than those ordinarily encountered in daily life or during the performance of routine physical or psychological examinations or tests."[10] This is frequently a difficult area of consideration for clinical research professionals. There can also be disagreement as to what presents risk in different populations.

Once an IRB has established that a proposed activity represents no more than minimal risk, two other questions must be considered: whether the proposed activity (1) falls within one of the 1998 categories (summarized above), or (2) represents a minor change in previously approved research. There is some room for interpretation on the latter. Different IRBs may have different assessments of what is considered a "minor change." Some IRBs have opted to carefully outline their understanding of "minor change" in their standard operating procedures (SOPs) or may include an algorithm that would help make the decision. This often helps avoid dispute when research activities are proposed.

An IRB might, for example, establish a list of proposed modifications in research activities that clearly do *not* qualify for expedited review. Entries on this list might include: (1) addition of a new drug, (2) addition of a new device, (3) addition of an invasive procedure, (4) increase in medication dose or a decrease in dose that may increase risk, (5) addition of vulnerable subjects to the study population, (6) prolongation of subjects' participation in the study other than for observational purpose, (7) changes in the inclusion/exclusion criteria that may involve incorporation of populations at greater risk, (8) identification of new, potentially significant risks, and (9) collection of additional blood samples that exceed the limits set in expedited category (2).

Protocol Amendments

It is common for research to be modified during the course of a clinical trial. Changes in previously approved research are referred to as "amendments" and must be submitted to an IRB in accordance with 21 *CFR* 56 and 45 *CFR* 46. Some amendments will qualify for expedited review as discussed in the preceding section of this chapter. Others will require full board review. Changes in approved research cannot be implemented without IRB approval unless the change is necessary to eliminate apparent immediate risks to subjects.[11] It is important to note that changes may include changes to the protocol, the informed consent document, advertising to recruit subjects, or other changes. Any change in a previously approved project or document must be reported to the IRB.

Continuing Review

Continuing review is often misunderstood. Continuing review must be substantive, meaningful, and occur at intervals no greater than once a year.[12] What is "substantive and meaningful continuing review"? The IRB should evaluate the following: (1) status of the study, (2) number of subjects enrolled during the approval period, (3) a summary of adverse events or unanticipated problems involving risks to subjects or others, (4) subjects' withdrawals, (5) complaints, (6) a summary of relevant recent literature if any, (7) findings obtained to date, (8) reports of data safety monitoring boards, and (9) a copy of the current approved informed consent document. Upon initial review of a new research proposal, an IRB should set a date when the research should be re-reviewed. The date should be based on the degree of risk involved in the study. IRBs need to clearly define this time point in their communications with investigators.

Many IRBs remind their investigators that a project is shortly due for continuing review. IRBs are not obligated to do this, but many do, as a service to their investigators. Investigators also should ensure that they track the time points and communicate appropriately with the IRB. If a project is not reconsidered at the assigned time, its IRB approval expires and research activities must cease. This emphasizes a recurrent theme throughout this text: various research entities must work together and each person or group (whether IRB, investigator, research coordinator, monitor, or sponsor) has a responsibility to protect subjects, follow the regulations and good clinical practice, and meet IRB expectations.

Dealing with Adverse Event Reports

Adverse event review is under the purview of the IRB and will be discussed further in chapter 4. It should be noted that The National Bioethics Advisory Commission's (NBAC's) recommendation number (5) suggested that the federal government create a uniform system for reporting and evaluating adverse events occurring in research, especially in multi-site research. NBAC's report stated, "The reporting and evaluation responsibilities of investigators, sponsors, institutional review boards, data safety monitoring boards, and federal agencies should be clear and efficient. The primary concern of the reporting system should be to protect current and prospective participants."[13]

2.4 PLANNING GENETIC RESEARCH THAT IS "IRB APPROVABLE"

Genetic testing and other tissue research has become crucial to the future of medicine, as it provides information that is important for the development of new treatments. Unfortunately, genetic information collected during research may have a negative impact on a subject's employability and insurability, should a breach of confidentiality occur. Further, the regulators offer little guidance.

Often a genetic sub-study may appear to be eligible for expedited review because "it's just an extra blood sample." IRBs generally determine that such sub-studies *do not* qualify for expedited review because of the potential risks inherent in genetic testing, such as breach of confidentiality, and the possible psychological or economic repercussions.

IRBs are expected to write and enforce policies to protect human subjects who participate in tissue collection studies. General concerns about breaches of privacy and confidentiality must be adequately addressed for an IRB to determine that genetic testing/tissue collection for research purposes is approvable.

To facilitate IRB review and approval, both the research protocol and the informed consent document should provide some additional information. Consent forms and protocols typically contain an introductory or background section; these should include a *general description of the genetic test* and an explanation of genetic testing and voluntary participation in terms understood by the subject. For example, this section might state,

> You are being asked to provide one [additional, if applicable] blood sample (about __ teaspoonfuls) for the study described below. You do not have to agree to be in this additional study in order to be in the main study of [name of study drug], if applicable.
>
> DNA is the material in your body's cells (genes) that pass on characteristics that are inherited from one generation to the next (like hair and eye color).
>
> DNA will be extracted from your blood sample in a laboratory so that your genetic information can be used to study [fill in].

Subjects continue to have a right to know the purpose of the research, including what information is expected to result from the research. This is increasingly difficult to convey in tissue research because investigators are not always able to predict what information may result from the study.

While *privacy* and *confidentiality* are required elements of informed consent and common elements in research protocols, they need to be taken a step further with a statement regarding identification of samples. For identified samples, the statement might read,

> Your sample will be identified by your subject number, or your name. To protect your privacy, only the investigator and the sponsor of the study, [name of sponsor], will be able to link your identity with your sample. Neither you nor your doctor will be given the results of the testing [when applicable].

For non-identified samples, the statement might read,

> Your sample will be given a number that cannot be linked with you. Your sample will be stored with thousands [or hundreds or many] other non-identified samples from [name of institution]. Since the sample cannot be linked to you, neither you nor your doctor will be given the results of the testing.

The risks of participating in a study should be clearly outlined to research subjects. It is important to note that there are frequently nonphysical risks. Additional information regarding risks to subjects and informed consent can be found in chapter 3. The following is sample language that might be useful in assuring a project's approvability with the IRB if the samples are identifiable.

> There is a chance of discrimination if the results of the testing show a genetic disorder. You might be denied a job or promotion, or denied health or life insurance if employers or insurance companies find out. You may experience other forms of discrimination. We will not release any information to anyone without your written permission. However, it is possible that genetic information may be gotten through legal means and affect your ability to get insurance or a job. In cases when parents and children are both tested, tests may reveal the possibility that the father is not the biological parent.

The potential benefits of genetic testing should also be considered, described in the protocol and in the consent form.

> This study may improve our understanding of the role of genes in [genetic condition]. Information learned about the gene may increase general knowledge, provide scientists with information about disease, and/or eventually lead to improved treatment. This will allow [or may allow] you to make informed healthcare decisions, but may be of no direct benefit to you or your family.

Concerns about Storage and Retrieval of Subjects' Samples

Investigators and sponsors must indicate whether subjects can retrieve their samples if they choose to discontinue their participation in the research. For example, a subject may request that his or her sample and data relating to study participation be destroyed at any time, but this would only be possible if the sample and data can be identified. Some state laws require that subjects be told how long the sample will be stored. In such cases, and when an investigator is not sure how/when he/she will use the specimens, it may be prudent to tell subjects that samples will be stored "indefinitely."

Consider how samples will be stored and what else might be done with them. The IRB should require that subjects either give written consent for additional testing for general research purposes, or that subjects give consent for no tests other than those described without additional permissions. A plan for storage and discard of samples should also be devised and outlined in both the protocol and the consent document. Particular attention should be paid when the investigator and/or sponsor use subjects' samples to create a cell line. Subjects should be asked if they are willing to have samples shared with investigators at the sponsor institution, at the same institution, at another institution, for the same or for different types of research.

Subjects cannot be asked to waive a legal right.[14] The term "donate" suggests abandonment of a legal right, and thus it is not generally considered acceptable language in an informed consent document of this nature. Finally, IRBs and sponsors may also be subject to state laws regarding genetic testing.

2.5 COMMON REASONS FOR IRB DEFERRAL, REJECTION, OR DELAY

An IRB has several options when it reviews proposed research. If an IRB determines that the criteria for approval have been met, a project can be "approved." When an IRB does not have sufficient information to make determinations, the project may be "deferred." Some protocols simply do not fulfill the human subjects protection requirements described earlier, and an IRB may be forced to reject these projects. If the requirements of approval are considered carefully during the design and preparation stage of a project, it is more likely to result in approval by the IRB.

In the wake of revisions to *The Declaration of Helsinki* in October 2000, some IRBs are deferring or rejecting protocols secondary to the questionable use of placebo arms. Item 29 of *The Declaration of Helsinki* states, "the benefits, risks, burdens, and effectiveness of a new method should be tested against those of the best current prophylactic, diagnostic and therapeutic methods. This does not exclude the use of placebo, or no treatment, in studies where no proven prophylactic, diagnostic or therapeutic method exists."[15]

Research proposals are also deferred or rejected when the approval criteria are unmet, or when there is a lack of clinical equipoise. *Clinical equipoise* refers to a genuine uncertainty on the part of the expert medical community about the comparative therapeutic merits of each arm of a clinical trial.[16]

Often the changes that an IRB requests be made to the informed consent document and/or protocol are substantive, and specific changes cannot be recommended during the convened meeting. In such cases deferral is necessary. The following is from OHRP's "Guidance on Written IRB Procedures" (2 April 2002):

> Convened IRBs often set conditions under which a protocol can be approved. OHRP recommends the following guidelines in such cases: only when the convened IRB stipulates specific revisions requiring simple concurrence by the investigators, may the IRB chair or another IRB member designated by the chair, subsequently approve the revised research protocol on behalf of the IRB under an expedited review procedure.[17]

IRB members are encouraged to review materials as far in advance of the meeting as possible, to address ethical or safety questions and concerns. When indicated, questions should be posed to the investigator, sponsor, or IRB consultant so that informed discussion can take place at the convened meeting. Clearly, this is not always possible and the purpose of a diverse membership is to ensure that different perspectives might identify different issues in subject safety and welfare. That being said, IRBs will defer research if they do not have enough information to comfortably approve or reject the proposed research.

Both investigators and sponsors should be responsive in addressing the IRB's questions after a deferral or rejection. A prompt and thorough response to a question or concern often leads to swift reconsideration by the committee and approval of the research. Most IRBs have policies that prescribe what an investigator should do in the event of deferral or rejection.

IRBs should clearly communicate their reasons for rejection or deferral. Investigators and sponsors should adequately address these concerns or questions if they intend to pursue IRB approval. IRBs should also provide as much information as possible, as quickly as is reasonable, to the IRB membership so that further review can take place before the meeting, fostering more informed discussion during the meeting. In an effort to be more efficient, some sponsors are now taking the time to meet with IRB administrators to develop informed consent templates that are acceptable to both the IRB and the sponsor.

2.6 SUGGESTIONS FOR AVOIDING DELAYS IN THE REVIEW PROCESS —IMPROVING EFFICIENCY WITHOUT SACRIFICING QUALITY OR INTEGRITY

Creative initiatives like the template consent document described above are key. Many investigational sites are organizing "super grants" departments or offices of clinical trials (recognizing the importance of establishing relationships with the key players in human subjects research). Some IRBs have developed standard language for risk and procedures, creating an efficient process for developing informed consent documents with nontechnical language. IRBs have improved their standard operating procedures, turning them into tools rather than simply rules to be followed.

As will be discussed in part E of chapter 8, numerous research suspensions at prestigious centers have led to an increase in educational opportunities for IRB members, staff, investigators, and other ancillary research staff. An encouraging trend is the increased focus on hiring additional qualified staff for the IRB.

Adherence to submission deadlines is another way to increase efficiency. The deadlines are established for a reason—to facilitate appropriate and timely review of materials.

Good clinical practice (GCP) auditors may ask investigators and IRBs why a policy is written a certain way. Often, a reasonable answer is not provided, but rather, "That is the way we've always done it." As the regulatory environment becomes increasingly complex, it is critical that IRB administrators and researchers revisit old ways of doing things in an effort to ensure that the IRB process is not cumbersome or inefficient.

Investigational sites are recognizing the value of regulatory affairs specialists who can help write consent forms and guide communications between investigators, sponsors, and the IRB. These groups collaborate with IRBs to develop research standards, tools to facilitate compliance, and quality improvement processes. Increased partnering with these departments will improve education and training of clinical research professionals, streamline review processes, and ensure that things get done correctly the first time.

Sponsors' changes to the consent document before and after the IRB meeting may contribute to delays. Sponsors should attempt to make only those changes that are substantive and do so as expeditiously as possible, with the understanding that the IRB has the final word on the informed consent document used at their research site.

2.7 THE IRB WANTS TO CHANGE THE PROTOCOL—IMPLICATIONS FOR MULTI-CENTER TRIALS

In some cases, an IRB may not be successful at effecting major changes in a multi-center protocol. It is likely that another IRB may have approved the very same project that the current IRB is proposing to reject. There are sometimes legitimate reasons for such discrepancies.

The FDA has proposed new legislation to prevent "IRB shopping." The proposal considers "whether to amend its [the FDA's] institutional review board (IRB) regulations to require sponsors and investigators to inform IRBs about any prior review decisions."[18] The change could prevent investigators and sponsors from ignoring one IRB's rejection/deferral and applying for review at another IRB. Numerous questions must be addressed before the FDA will consider drafting a regulation. Nonetheless, this may be another opportunity to increase communication in the clinical research community.

2.8 EFFECTIVELY AND TACTFULLY MANAGING WHAT LOOKS LIKE IRB "NITPICKING"

In 2001, Independent Review Consulting, Inc. (IRC) published a calendar with cartoons by Don Mayne.[19] One was a picture of an IRB sitting at a round table, each member turned toward the person next to them, picking for nits in their neighbor member's hair. IRBs do "nitpick." It is their job, in part, to do so. The obligation to preserve the safety and welfare of human research subjects is an enormous one. Many IRBs are further concerned with ensuring that the research proposal and the conduct of are the best that they can be. This often means detailed attention to items that may seem minor to those trying to get through "the system." As stated in the previous section, "nitpicking" by sponsors can also contribute to delays in IRB approval.

2.9 HOW CAN SPONSORS AND INVESTIGATORS NAVIGATE THE IRB REVIEW PROCESS?

Get It Right the First Time

Sponsors and investigators should ensure that multiple reviews of the protocol and consent form are performed before they ever get to an IRB. While a team approach may seem to slow down progress in some settings, several readers are generally better than one at catching errors and omissions.

View Requests for Changes as Constructive

Investigators, sponsors, and IRBs are all on a learning curve, discovering new and improved ways to protect human subjects. Keep up with the trends. Join listservs (see the section "Useful Websites" at the end of this book) to keep current on what's happening in the human subjects protection arena. Respect the IRB's expertise. The IRB is in the business of protecting subjects, and sometimes that means asking questions (thus causing delays), while the committee ensures that it is fulfilling its ethical and legal responsibilities. Investigators need to follow the IRB's policies, keep on the pulse of what's happening in the human subjects protection arena, and consult with the IRB before submission.

2.10 WHAT CAN THE IRB DO TO FACILITATE REVIEW?

The IRB can also help. Clearly written, current standard operating procedures may address many questions that may arise. Train members to have a discriminating eye. Encourage them to review things as much in advance of the meeting as possible in order to identify questions that can be answered early in the process.

Cut to the chase—communicate with the sponsor directly when there are disputes or concerns. This is discussed further in chapter 8, "Especially for IRB Staff." Invite investigators and other research staff to IRB meetings so that they can observe first hand the purpose, the process, and mechanisms of the IRB.

2.11 TAKE AWAY MESSAGES

- The requirements for IRB approval are grounded in the basic principles of the National Commission's 1979 *Belmont Report.*
- Consider the "approvability" requirements when a protocol is being written and designed and you are more likely to yield an approvable protocol.
- The basic difference between full review and expedited review is that full review must take place at a convened meeting of an IRB.
- Be familiar with regulations and standard operating procedures of the IRB
- Respect IRB submission deadlines.
- Continuing review must be substantive and meaningful, and occur at no greater intervals than once per year.

- Both investigators and sponsors should be responsive in addressing an IRB's questions after a deferral or rejection. A prompt and thorough response to a question or concern frequently leads to swift reconsideration by the committee and approval of the research.

NOTES

1. Department of Health, Education and Welfare, *The Belmont Report* (Washington, D.C.: U.S. Government Printing Office, 1988, 201/778-80319 GPO 887-809); originally published in 44 Federal Register (18 April 1979), 23192-7; *http://ohrp.osophs.dhhs.gov/human subjects/guidance/belmont.htm*, accessed 10 July 2002.

2. 21 *CFR* 56.111; 45 *CFR* 46.111.

3. 21 *CFR* 56.111(a)(6); 45 *CFR* 46.111 (a)(6); *Belmont*, see note 1 above.

4. 21 *CFR* 56.111(a)(1); 45 *CFR* 46.111 (a)(1).

5. 21 *CFR* 56.111(a)(2); 45 *CFR* 46.111 (a)(2).

6. 21 *CFR* 56.111(a)(3), 45 *CFR* 46.111 (a)(3)

7. 21 *CFR* 56.111; 45 *CFR* 46.111.

8. 21 *CFR* 56.108(c); 21 *CFR* 56.110, 45 *CFR* 46.108(b), 45 *CFR* 46.110.

9. *Categories of Research that May Be Reviewed by the Institutional Review Board (IRB) through an Expedited Review Procedure*, *http://ohrp.osophs.dhhs.gov/humansubjects/guidance/expedited98.htm*, accessed 22 May 2002.

10. 45 *CFR* 46.102(l); 21 *CFR* 50.3(k) and 56.102(j).

11. 21 *CFR* 312.66; ICH GCP Guideline 4.5.2; ICH GCP Guidelines—E6, *http://www.ifpma.org/pdf>ifpma/e6.pdf*, accessed 28 May 2002.

12. 21 *CFR* 56.109(f), 45 *CFR* 46.109(e); ICH GCP Guidelines 3.1.4, see note 11 above.

13. National Bioethics Advisory Commission (NBAC), *Ethical and Policy Issues in Research Involving Human Participants*, *http://bioethics.georgetown. edu/nbac/human/oversumm.pdf, accessed 26 June 2002.*

14. Office for Protection from Research Risks, *Exculpatory Language in Informed Consent Documents*, 15 November 1996, *http://ohrp.osophs.dhhs.gov/humansubjects/guidance/exculp.htm*, accessed 1 July 2002.

15. World Medical Association, *The Declaration of Helsinki* (1964, revised 1975, 1983, 1989), *http://ohsr.od.nih.gov/helsinki.php3*, accessed 15 February 2003.

16. OHRP, "Considerations of Research Design: Section H, Clinical Trials," in *Institutional Review Board Guidebook*, chap. 4, *http://ohrp.osophs.dhhs.gov/irb/irb_chapter4.htm*, accessed 2 July 2002.

17. OHRP, *Guidance on Written IRB Procedures*, 2 April 2002, *http://ohrp.osophs.dhhs.gov/humansubjects/guidance/wirbproc.pdf*, accessed 1 July 2002.

18. "Proposed Rules," 21 *CFR* 56; "Institutional Review Boards: Requiring Sponsors and Investigators to Inform IRBs of Any Prior Reviews," Docket No. 01N-0322, *Federal Register*, 67, no. 44 (6 March 2002): 10115-6.

19. Cartoon by Don Mayne, *IRB Calendar*, 2001 (San Anselmo, Calif.: Independent Review Consulting, 2001, *http://www.irb-irc.net.*

3

Consent Issues

Kimberly Irvine, BS

This chapter will address various informed consent issues as they affect research sponsors and investigational sites. It will provide tips and suggestions about how to approach writing an informed consent document.

Issues to be considered include:

3.1 What Is the Process of Informed Consent?
3.2 The Elements of Informed Consent Forms
3.3 Exculpatory Language
3.4 Financial Disclosure and Conflicts of Interest
3.5 Assent in Child Subjects and Sample Consent Form
3.6 Sample HIPAA Authorization Form
3.7 Consent for Sub-Studies
3.8 Sample Consent Form for Genetic Testing and/or Tissue Banking
3.9 Sponsors' Considerations
3.10 Common Problems with Consent Form Templates Received from Study Sponsors
3.11 Take Away Messages

This chapter is designed to provide some practical tips and guidance for creating an informed consent document that is understandable to subjects, meets the regulations of the U.S. Food and Drug Administration (FDA), the Office for Human Research Protections (OHRP), and the Health Insurance Portability and Accountability Act (HIPAA), and increases the chances of approval by an institutional review board (IRB).

The process of informed consent is a human rights issue, and is based on the fundamental principles of "respect for others." Documents such as *The Nuremberg Code,*[1] *The Belmont Report,*[2] and *The Declaration of Helsinki*[3] are basic to the development of what is now termed the *process of informed consent.*

3.1 WHAT IS THE PROCESS OF INFORMED CONSENT?

The informed consent process must take place prior to any involvement of a subject in a research trial. Subjects may voluntarily decide to participate in research only after being fully informed of all associated procedures and their potential risks and benefits. It is the responsibility of the principal investigator to ensure that all information is provided in writing as well as orally and at a comprehension level that can be readily understood.

The regulations anticipate that there will be an oral exchange of information between the investigator and the subject as part of this process. This too must be given in speech understandable to the subject. Additionally, if English is not the subject's native language, translated versions (IRB approved) of the consent document should be available and a translator should be present to confer with the subject. The investigator should encourage and respond to any questions the subject may have. It is important that it be clear to investigators and subjects that there are differences between obtaining consent and the informed consent document. The informed consent document should serve as a guide to what will happen during the course of the study.

Thus, informed consent should be regarded as the process that takes place between the subject and the principal investigator or a member of the study staff, during which the specifics of the study are discussed. The informed consent discussion should last until both the subject and the person obtaining consent feel confident that the trial has been satisfactorily described and the subject has a reasonable understanding of the consequences of his or her participation. Potential subjects must be given ample opportunity to consider whether or not they want to participate in a research study. In addition to the informed consent discussion, it is desirable, whenever possible, to give the prospective participant sufficient time to review the document and discuss it with family and friends. The documentation of the consent process should be in writing and signed and dated by the subject or the subject's legally authorized representative (depending on state and/or institutional policy regarding substitute consent).[4]

The individual obtaining consent from the subject should sign and date the informed consent document. A copy should be given to the subject or the surrogate and the original should be maintained with the investigator's research records. Additionally, if the subject is an in-patient, some institutions require that a copy of the consent be placed in the medical record.

The Risk of Coercion

People are often vulnerable when they discuss health problems with their doctor. They may want to please their caretaker and may agree to whatever their physician suggests. It is very important that the investigator minimize the possibility of coercion or undue influence.

Keep It Simple

Consent forms should be written in nonscientific, simple terms that research subjects can readily understand. The consent form should be written at the comprehension level of a sixth grader. This can be challenging for medical professionals. The more familiar one is with medical terminology, the more difficult it becomes to reduce these terms to lay language. A glossary of some commonly used medical terms and some procedures, abstracted from the Mount Sinai School of Medicine and the Biomedical Research Alliance of New York's (BRANY's) IRB procedures, can be found at the end of this book. Other suggestions to improve the readability of the informed consent document include:

- Prepare the consent document using a 12-point font.
- Avoid run-on sentences and keep sentences and paragraphs short and to the point.
- Use headings to identify new topics and bullets.

- Avoid the use of both the medical term and a lay definition— for example, insomnia (difficulty sleeping or falling asleep), nausea (upset stomach), anorexia (loss of appetite)—as this is more difficult to follow. When in doubt, use the lay definition.
- Use proper grammar and punctuation.
- Many IRBs suggest the use of the word "subject" when referring to a research study participant. A patient-doctor relationship is different from a subject-investigator relationship. The word "subject" helps clarify that the discussion is about "research."
- Avoid lengthy consent forms, as long forms may affect comprehension.

What is the Goal?

When developing the informed consent document, keep in mind that the ultimate goal is to provide the potential subject with all the information needed to make an *informed* decision about participation in the research trial.

3.2 THE ELEMENTS OF INFORMED CONSENT FORMS

The U.S. Department of Health and Human Services (DHHS), at 45 *CFR* 46 Subpart A, and the *Code of Federal Regulations* (*CFR*), at 21 *CFR* 50 and 21 *CFR* 56 (hereafter referred to as the "Common Rule"), require that certain information be provided to research subjects before they participate in a study.[5] In addition, the Privacy Rule, established as part of the Health Insurance Portability and Accountability Act of 1996 (HIPAA) legislation, affects many areas of healthcare, including research.[6] Specifically, human subjects must authorize the use or disclosure of their protected health information (PHI).

Obtaining written authorization from a research subject is one of several ways that researchers can access and use PHI. The Privacy Rule outlines other pathways that investigators can use to collect information, including the following:

- Access information that is de-identified.
- Obtain a waiver of authorization from a privacy board.
- Access information for review prior to beginning the conduct of research.
- Use a limited data set that restricts the use of certain subject identifiers.
- Review the PHI of the deceased, which does not require authorization.

Some organizations use an IRB-approved consent and attach a HIPAA-compliant authorization form. Others incorporate HIPAA requirements into the consent form. IRB approval may not be required for the separate authorization form, but policy on this varies from organization to organization. Check with your organization's privacy officer for your organization's policy.

The following is a list of elements required by the "Common Rule." Examples will be given that incorporate language that is applicable to and compliant with both the "Common Rule" and HIPAA legislation.

12 Elements of Informed Consent from the "Common Rule"

Element 1: A Statement that the Study Involves Research[7]

Example

You are being asked to participate in a research project because you have been diagnosed with high blood pressure.

Common Errors and Omissions

- Failure to include the reason the subject is considered a candidate for the study. The statement "You are being invited to participate in a research trial" or something similar is inadequate.

- Use of the word "invite." This should be replaced with "asked." People are "invited" to parties, not to a research trial.
- Inclusion of the inclusion and exclusion criteria for the study. It is the investigator's responsibility to determine whether or not a subject is eligible for participation. The subject should not have to make this determination.

Element 2: An Explanation of the Purposes of the Research[8]

Example

> The primary purpose of this study is to compare the effectiveness and safety of experimental drug, XX, which has not yet been approved for use by the U.S. Food and Drug Administration (FDA), with that of an FDA-approved drug called YY.

Common Errors and Omissions

- Use of terms like "new" instead of "experimental" or "investigational" to describe the status of the study drug. Words like "new" may be perceived as describing a drug that has been "approved" by the FDA. The word "experimental" emphasizes the point that this is research.
- Omission of the definition of an "experimental" drug,[9] that is:

  > An experimental drug has not yet been approved for use by the U.S. Food and Drug Administration.

- Writing the informed consent document in the "wrong" person. Many but not all IRBs require that consent forms should be written as if the person obtaining consent is presenting it to the subject. The FDA recommends that the consent form be written in the second person ("You/your" instead of "I/my"). Find out what the IRB requires.
- Use of the phrase "You understand." When possible, delete words and phrases that reference what subjects are expected to understand.[10] Instead, use clear statements, such as the following examples:

  > Your participation in this study is voluntary.

  or

  > You may withdraw from this study at any time without penalty or loss of benefits to which you are otherwise entitled.

  The consent document must not put subjects in the position of certifying that the information they have received is complete. Avoid using statements such as "You understand all of procedures and risks involved in this study." Instead, try:

  > You have had an opportunity to review this consent form and have all of your questions answered to your satisfaction.

- Neglecting to review the protocol to ensure the study objectives are reflected in the consent form. Often the rationale for the study is not clearly stated.

Element 3: The Expected Duration of the Subjects' Participation[11]

Example

> Your participation in this study will last 6 weeks.

Common Errors and Omissions

- Forgetting to inform the subjects of how long their expected participation in the entire study will take.

Element 4: A Description of the Procedures to Be Followed[12]

Guidance and Sample Language

- A description of every visit and procedure must be addressed in the consent form, including, but not limited to, blood draws, electrocardiograms (EKGs), injections, follow-up phone calls, pulmonary function testing, x-rays, or any other procedure done in accordance with the protocol. Even completion of questionnaires, diaries, or postcards must be included in the consent document. To ensure that all procedures are accounted for, the author of the consent document should compare the procedures listed on the consent form to those described in the protocol.

  With respect to drawing blood, it is important to include the amount of blood to be drawn, for example:

  > Approximately 7 tablespoons of blood will be drawn during the course of the study.

  The amount of blood should be described in measurements of teaspoons or tablespoons (5 ml = 1 teaspoon, 15 ml = 1 tablespoon). Most subjects have a better idea of the liquid volume of a teaspoon or tablespoon than they do of a cc (cubic centimeter) or of a ml (milliliter). Note: A blood count tube is approximately 7 ml (.5 tablespoon) and a serum chemistry tube is approximately 10 ml (2 teaspoons).
- If the study requires subjects to be "randomized" or "randomly assigned," this process must be explained to the subject in the consent form. Common phrases that can be used to describe randomization may include:

  - like the flip of a coin [when the chances are 50/50]

  or

  - by chance
  - like a lottery
  - like the roll of the dice
  - like picking chances from a hat.

- The dosage of the study drug to be administered to the subject should be included in this section of the consent form.[13]

  > If you are randomized to receive drug XX, you will receive one of the following doses: 300 mg per day, 600 mg per day, or 900 mg per day. Your chances of receiving placebo are 1 in 4.

- Is the study double-blinded? This too must be explained.

  > Neither you nor the investigator will know which treatment you receive. In the event of an emergency, your investigator can determine which drug you are receiving.

- Does the protocol require a washout period? This process must be explained to the patient:

  > A period of time in which you will be asked not to take your current medication.

- Is the study open-label, placebo controlled, or evaluator blinded? These phrases are not lay language and need to be described.
- The consent form should address the duration of individual visits and procedures, including questionnaires.

Common Errors and Omissions

- Omission of the length of time associated with procedures, visits, and so on. Include estimates of the time that will be needed, such as:

> The quality of life questionnaire will take about 30 minutes to complete.
>
> or
>
> Study visit 2 will take approximately 1 hour.

Element 5: Identification of Any Procedures that Are Experimental[14]

Guidance and Sample Language

Procedures that are considered experimental must be identified as such:

> Placing a catheter into the artery to open it up is an alternative to surgery, but is considered experimental.

Common Errors and Omissions

- Listing only "experimental" procedures in the informed consent. All procedures and visits that occur during the protocol must be addressed in the consent. Procedures that are not simply part of clinical care but are required as part of the research must still be described in the consent.
- Failure to distinguish between standard of care and experimental procedures.

Element 6: Description of Any Reasonably Foreseeable Risks or Discomforts to the Subject[15]

Guidance and Sample Language

> The reported side-effects of study drug XX were generally mild and short-term. The side-effects reported most frequently include cough, headache, dizziness, and sore throat. These are generally reversible. Rarely, side-effects such as swelling of the face, lips, hands, or feet, and allergic reaction have occurred.
>
> You will be asked to discontinue any current treatment for your high blood pressure, including prescribed medications or herbal therapy, for the duration of the study. If you stop your antihypertensives, your blood pressure may increase and increase your risk of stroke or cardiovascular events. . . . If your condition does not improve or worsens, you should contact the investigator immediately.
>
> You may be given placebo, an inactive substance, during the study. If you receive placebo, your condition may go untreated and may worsen as a result.
>
> The radiation you receive from the chest x-ray is minimal. The more radiation you receive over the course of your life, however, the greater the risk of inducing changes to the cells in your body or of having cancerous tumors. The changes to your body's cells possibly could cause abnormalities or disease in your future offspring. The radiation from this study is not expected to greatly increase these risks, but the exact increase in such risks is not known.
>
> Risks and discomforts associated with drawing blood samples may include pain, bruising, light-headedness, and, on rare occasions, infection.
>
> The study drug must only be taken by the person for whom it has been prescribed and must be kept out of the reach of children and persons who have a limited capacity to read or understand.

Common Errors and Omissions

- Omission of the risks of drugs used as part of the research plan even if they are approved agents. The risks of all drugs used during the study (including placebo) must be disclosed in the consent document.
- Failure to include the risks associated with procedures listed in the protocol. Procedures such as x-rays, placement

of an intravenous line, venipuncture, colonoscopy, bronchoscopy, and others all carry risks which should be included in the risk section of the informed consent.

- Failure to address the availability of the study drug to the subject once the study is over. Some IRBs require that subjects must be informed whether or not the study drug will be available to them once their participation in the study is over.
- Omission of risks associated with stopping or withdrawing from the subject's current medications (washout period).
- Description of risks in medical terms instead of lay terminology (for example, orthostatic hypotension, respiratory depression, bradycardia, and tinnitus).
- Referring to a risk as an "adverse event." It is preferable to use terms such as "side-effect" or "bad effect."
- Failure to "cross check" the procedure section against the risk section to identify omissions in one or both areas.

Pregnant Women

Guidance and Sample Language[16]

> There may be unforeseen risks to an unborn child associated with your taking drug XX. For this reason, you must agree to use a highly effective means of birth control, such as hormonal contraceptives, intrauterine device (IUD), an implantable contraceptive (such as Norplant), an injectable contraceptive (Depo-Provera), a barrier method of contraception (such as a condom or diaphragm with spermicide) or abstinence. You should discuss your methods of birth control with the study doctor. You must notify the study doctor if you suspect that you may be pregnant or if you are a male and suspect your partner may be pregnant.
>
> The effects of drug XX on a nursing infant are unknown; if you are breast-feeding, you cannot participate in the study.

Common Errors and Omissions

- Failure to make reference to males in consideration of their partners.
- Not listing the specific methods of birth control required by the protocol.
- Not informing the subject that some drugs may interact with hormonal contraceptives and render them ineffective.

Element 7: A Description of Any Benefits to the Subject or to Others that May Reasonably be Expected from the Research[17]

Example

> Participation in this study may help to improve your condition, but it is also possible that your condition may worsen. There is no guarantee that you will personally benefit by participating in this research study. Your participation in this study may provide information that may help other people who have a similar medical problem in the future.

Common Errors and Omissions

- Listing payment, free medication, and/or close monitoring of "your condition" as benefits of study participation. Such information placed here could be considered coercive, and is better located in the "cost" or "reimbursement" section of the consent document.
- Omission of a statement such as, "There is no guarantee that you will benefit from study participation."

Element 8: A Disclosure of Appropriate Alternative Procedures or Courses of Treatment, If Any, that Might Be Available to the Subject[18]

Guidance and Sample Language

> You do not have to participate in this research study to receive treatment for your

condition. You may choose not to be in this study. This will not jeopardize your care in any way. There are other drugs such as XX, YY, or ZZ that your doctor can prescribe to treat your condition. The investigator will discuss alternative treatments with you.

- Alternative medications that may treat the condition under study should be included.
- Subjects must be told that they will be treated for their condition even if they refuse to participate in research. Subjects should be advised of their options.
- If indicated, inform subjects that there are no alternatives to participation; there may be alternative palliative treatments that are not curative. This information should be shared with subjects.
- If the drug used in the study is FDA approved, subjects should be informed that the study drug is commercially available and they do not have to participate in the research study to have access to the agent under study.

Common Errors and Omissions

- Failure to inform subjects that one alternative would be not to participate in the research study.
- Omission of a listing of the other medications or classes of drugs that are available to treat a subject's condition. A statement such as, "Other drugs are available to treat your condition and the investigator will discuss these alternatives with you," is not very informative. It is often helpful to include brand names if generic names are used.

Element 9: A Statement Describing the Extent, If Any, to which Confidentiality of Records Identifying the Subject Will Be Maintained[19]

The requirements mandated by HIPAA may be incorporated into the body of the consent form or can be addressed in a separate document (see Figure 3.6). Under HIPAA requirements, subjects must authorize the use of their protected health information (PHI). The confidentiality section of the informed consent form is an appropriate place to incorporate some of the privacy language that is required by HIPAA. Other sections in this chapter contain sample language that is relevant to HIPAA.[20] In these sections, the HIPAA text is presented in **bold print.**

Guidance and Sample Language

Your medical records will be kept as confidential as possible within the limitations of state and federal law. **Federal privacy regulations require that you authorize the release of any health information that may reveal your identity. The persons and entities that you are authorizing to use or disclose your individually identifiable health information may include the study doctor, the study staff, the institution, the sponsor, and [list all applicable parties]. In order to analyze the data collected during this research study,** all of the health information generated or collected about you during this study may be inspected by the study sponsor or the authorized agents of the sponsor, the FDA, the Department of Health and Human Services (DHHS) agencies, the institutional review board, and governmental agencies in other countries **[list other parties as appropriate].** Because of the need to release information to these parties, absolute confidentiality cannot be guaranteed.

Once your personal health information is released it may be redisclosed, at which point your health information will no longer be protected by federal privacy regulations. The results of this research may be presented at meetings or in publications; however, your identity will not be disclosed in those presentations. By signing this informed consent form, you are authorizing such access to your medical records. **This authorization will have no expiration. [Or: This authorization will expire on month/day/year.]**

HIPAA-Required Elements

- **Description of information to be used or disclosed.**
- **Persons authorized to use and disclose information.**
- **Persons authorized to receive information.**
- **Purpose of the requested use or disclosure of information.**
- **Redisclosure of information.**
- **Expiration of authorization.**

Common Errors and Omissions

- Failure to inform subjects of all the parties that will have access to their medical and study records (sponsors, sponsors' representatives, IRB auditors, FDA representatives, and other governmental agencies from countries where the study drug may be considered for approval).
- Failure to inform subjects that by signing the consent form they are giving permission for these agencies and representatives to review their records.
- Not clearly stating that absolute confidentiality cannot be guaranteed.

Element 10: Statement Addressing the Availability of Compensation If Injury Occurs as a Result of Participation in the Study[20]

Guidance and Sample Language

- Sample clauses addressing compensation for injury:

  If you suffer an illness or injury from the study drug or from properly performed study procedures, the sponsor will cover the medical expenses necessary to treat such illness or injury to the extent not covered by insurance or a government program. No other compensation will be offered by the sponsor or the institution. By signing this form, you are not waiving any legal right to seek additional compensation through the courts.

or

  If you are injured as a result of your participation in this study, immediate, short-term medical care will be made available to you. The costs of such medical care will be billed to you or your insurance company or government program. No other compensation will be offered. You are not waiving any legal rights by signing this form.[21]

- The sponsor will usually provide language that details what costs it will cover in case illness or injury arise as a result of a subject's participation in the study. It should not include statements such as, "Sponsor will not pay for expenses that are attributable to the negligence or misconduct of the investigator or the institution." Such language may be considered exculpatory, as it appears to ask subjects to release the sponsor from certain liabilities. Moreover, *negligence* is a legal term that subjects cannot be expected to understand. Subjects who participate in research have the same rights as others to seek compensation for an injury, and consent forms should not infer otherwise.
- Other acceptable language:

  Only costs in excess of what is paid for by your insurance or other government program will be reimbursed.

If applicable, the consent form must clearly state,

  No other compensation will be offered by the sponsor or institution.

- The compensation for injury clause should also include some reference to the subject's rights:

  You are not giving up any of your legal rights by signing this form.

or

  You are not waiving your legal right to seek additional compensation by signing this form.[22]

The informed consent document must clearly state what form of compensation for injury is available to the subject. If no compensation is available, plainly say so. There is no requirement to discuss compensation that is *not* available.

Common Errors and Omissions

- Avoid the use of exculpatory language. For example, avoid "No compensation is available," and "You will be responsible," or "The sponsor will not be responsible."
- Do not omit this entire section. If compensation for injury is not available to subjects, the section should still be included in the document. Note: If the research is deemed minimal risk, there is no requirement to include language regarding compensation for injury, but many institutions/sponsors/IRBs still include this section.
- Use of complex legal terminology.
- Failure to include a statement explaining that subjects do not waive any legal rights. Statements made about subjects' rights are sometimes ambiguous. Often we will see the following language in the consent, "You are not waiving any of your rights as a research subject by signing this consent form." This sentence may lead subjects to believe that, as research subjects, their rights differ from the rights of those not participating in a research study.

Element 11: An Explanation of Whom to Contact with Questions about the Research Study, Research-Related Injury, or Research Subjects' Rights[23]

Examples

> If you have any questions concerning your participation in this study, or if you feel you have experienced a research-related injury or a reaction to the study medication, you should contact Dr. Mary Smith at [include phone number], the principal investigator.
>
> If you have any questions about your rights as a research subject, you may contact the institutional review board at [include phone number here].

- The consent form must indicate whom subjects should contact if they have any questions about the study, their rights as research subjects, or if they think they have suffered an injury as a result of participating in the study.

Common Errors and Omissions

- Incorrect phone numbers. One wrong digit may result in subjects being unable to reach help when they have questions or side-effects.

Element 12: Statement Indicating that Participation Is Voluntary, Refusal to Participate Will Involve No Penalty or Loss of Benefits to which the Subject Is Otherwise Entitled, and the Subject May Discontinue Participation at any Time without Penalty or Loss of Benefits to which the Subject Is Otherwise Entitled[24]

Guidance and Sample Language

> Your participation in this research study is voluntary. You have the right to decline participation or to withdraw from this study at

any time. This will in no way affect your current or future medical care.

[You may also revoke the authorization to use or disclose personal information about your health. If you chose to withdraw your authorization, you must notify the study doctor in writing. The study doctor's mailing address is [provide address]. The study doctor will still be able to use the information collected about you prior to your withdrawal from the study. Information that has already been sent to the study sponsor cannot be withdrawn.]*

HIPAA-Required Element

- Subjects must know that their participation in a study is completely voluntary and they can choose to withdraw from the study at any time without penalty or loss of benefits to which they would otherwise be entitled.[25] If a subject withdraws, he or she should not be jeopardizing his or her relationship with the investigator, or the subject's physician (if different).
- **Subjects must be informed that they can withdraw their authorization to allow the release of any of their individually identifiable health information. However, information that has already been disclosed cannot be withdrawn. It is also important to emphasize that this request must be submitted in writing to the principal investigator.**

Elements of the Informed Consent Form Recommended by ICH

The *Code of Federal Regulations* refers to six "additional" elements of informed consent, to be included when appropriate. The International Conference on Harmonisation (ICH) recommends that these elements be included in all consent forms. These six elements follow.

Element 1: Statement that the Particular Treatment or Procedure May Involve Risks to the Subject that Are Currently Unforeseeable[26]

Example

There may be risks or side-effects related to the study drug that are unknown at this time. You will be notified of any significant new findings become known that may affect your willingness to continue in the study.

Common Errors and Omissions

- Failure to include this section in the consent form.

Element 2: Anticipated Circumstances under which the Subject's Participation May Be Terminated by the Investigator without regard to the Subject's Consent[27]

Example

Your participation in this study may be discontinued without your consent by the investigator or the sponsoring company if you fail to follow the investigator's instructions. You may also be withdrawn from the study if, in the investigator's or sponsor's opinion, the study drug is ineffective, harmful, or has medically unacceptable side-effects, or for other reasons at the discretion of the sponsor or investigator. If you are withdrawn from the study, you will be asked to have appropriate medical tests and follow up to evaluate your health and safety.

* If the research institution, IRB, or privacy board requires the use of a separate authorization form, this paragraph does not need to be included in the consent form.

Common Errors and Omissions

- Inclusion of a vague blanket statement that subjects may be withdrawn from the study at any time. Subjects must be advised of the possible reasons for withdrawal by the investigator or the sponsor.

Element 3: Any Additional Costs to Subjects that May Result from Participation in the Research[28]

Guidance and Sample Language

- Subjects must be informed of any additional costs that they may incur that are related to participation in the study. If there are no additional costs, the consent form must state this: "There will be no additional cost to you for participation in this research trial," or "The study drug will be provided at no cost to you."
- If the subjects' insurance is to be billed for procedures and visits that are part of the research, subjects must be so informed.
- If there is reimbursement for subjects' travel expenses or any other compensation to subjects, the dollar amount should be clearly defined and an explanation of proration, if any, should be clear.
- Subjects should be informed about how and when they will receive such reimbursement.

You will be reimbursed a maximum of $150 for your participation in this study to help offset the cost of your time and travel to the investigator's office. If your participation in the study ends prior to study completion, you will be reimbursed $25 for each study visit you completed. Such reimbursement will be made by check four to six weeks after each completed study visit.

- Subjects' reimbursement should not be excessive, as it may be considered coercive. Usually subjects receive between $25 and $50 for each outpatient visit. Unusually long visits or procedures may carry higher reimbursement. Investigators are encouraged to check their IRB's reimbursement guidelines. Ordinarily, subjects would not receive any compensation for in-patient studies unless they are being admitted to the hospital solely for the research trial or when an outpatient follow-up visit is mandatory.

Common Errors and Omissions

- Failure to disclose if the reimbursement will be prorated if subjects do not complete the study.
- Including information in the "Compensation for Injury" section about additional costs to the subject. "Costs" and "Compensation for Injury" should be two separate and distinct sections of the informed consent document.
- Offering excessive reimbursement that can raise the possibility of coercion.
- Not informing subjects about when and in what form they will be compensated.

Element 4: The Consequences of a Subject's Decision to Withdraw from Research and Procedures for Orderly Termination of Participation by the Subject[29]

Example

If you decide to withdraw from this research study, you must inform the investigator. For safety reasons, you will be asked to return to the clinic for a final study visit.

Common Errors and Omissions

- Not including a statement that instructs any subjects who do not finish the study that it may be in their best interest to return to the clinic for a final visit.

- Suggesting that subjects *must* return for a final visit.

Element 5: Statement that Significant New Findings Developed during the Course of the Research that May Relate to the Subject's Willingness to Continue Will Be Provided to the Subject[30]

Guidance and Sample Language

You will be notified of any significant new findings that may affect your willingness to continue in the study.

- This statement can usually be found at the end of the "Risks" section.

Element 6: Approximate Number of Subjects Involved in the Study[31]

Guidance and Sample Language

Approximately 75 subjects will participate in this research study.

- A statement of this nature may usually be found in one of two sections in the consent form, either the "Introduction" or the "Purpose of the Study."

Common Errors and Omissions

- Failure to list the number of subjects expected to participate in the study.

Additional Elements of Informed Consent

The following three elements should also be included in informed consent forms.

Additional Element 1: Treatment and the Probability of Random Assignment to Placebo or Treatment Arms

Guidance and Sample Language

- The chances of receiving the study drug versus placebo should be documented in the consent form, for example, "Your chances of receiving the study drug are 50/50."
- When applicable, this element is typically found in the "Procedures" section of the consent document, where the process of randomization is identified.

Common Errors and Omissions

- Failing to include the subject's chances of receiving the study drug versus another agent or agents.
- Inaccurately describing the chances, such as "like the flip of a coin" when the chances are not 50/50.

Additional Element 2: Statement of Consent

This is another section of the consent in which HIPAA-related language might be incorporated into the body of the consent.*

Sample Language

You have read the above description of this research study. You have been informed of the risks and benefits involved and all your questions have been answered to your satisfaction. By signing this form, you voluntarily consent to participate in the research study.

Unless you authorize the use and disclosure of your personal health information,

* If the research institution, IRB, or privacy board requires the use of a separate authorization form, this paragraph does not need to be included in the consent form.

you cannot participate in this research study. If you refuse to give your authorization your medical care will not be affected.

Right of Refusal

- Typically there is a short consent statement at the end of the document where subjects are asked to confirm that they have read the consent form, their questions have been answered satisfactorily, and they voluntarily agree to participate in the study, acknowledge that they are not waiving any legal rights, and authorize release of their medical records.
- There should be a statement here that states, "You will receive a copy of this consent form for your records."

Additional Element 3: Signatures

Guidelines on who must sign the informed consent form vary, depending on the state, IRB, and institutional requirements. Requested signatures may include: the subject or the subject's legally authorized representative, the principal investigator, the person obtaining consent, and/ or a witness. Federal policy only requires the signature of the subject or the subject's legally authorized representative when using a standard informed consent document. A witness is not required. Also, there is no requirement that a subject must initial each page of the consent form. A minimal requirement of most IRBs is a signature by the person obtaining the informed consent.

3.3 EXCULPATORY LANGUAGE

The consent form should not contain exculpatory language. Within the context of informed consent, exculpatory language can be defined as *words or phrases that ask or appear to ask a subject to waive or give up his or her legal rights.* Exculpatory language may also include *asking subjects to release the investigators, sponsors, or institutions from liability for negligence or willful misconduct.* Avoid using statements that require subjects to agree to terms or conditions, as this can be construed as being exculpatory (for example, "I agree that I will not be paid for any research related injuries.") Stick to accurate statements, such as, "You will not be offered payment for any research-related injuries."

Examples of Exculpatory Language

- "By agreeing to this use, you should understand that you would give up all claims to personal benefit from commercial or other use of these substances."
- "I voluntarily and freely donate any and all blood, urine, and tissue and hereby relinquish all right, title, and interest to said items."
- "By consenting to participate in this research, I give up any property rights I may have to the bodily fluids or tissue samples obtained in the course of the research."
- "I waive any possibility of compensation for injuries that I may receive as a result of participation in this research."

Examples of Acceptable Language

Tissue obtained from you in this research may be used to establish a cell line that could be patented and licensed. There are no plans to provide financial compensation to you should this occur.

By consenting to participate, you authorize the use of your bodily fluids and tissue samples for the research described above.

This hospital is not able to offer financial compensation nor to absorb the costs of medical treatment should you be injured as a result of participating in this research.

> This hospital makes no commitment to provide free medical care or payment for any unfavorable outcomes resulting from participation in this research. Medical services will be offered at the usual charge.[32]

3.4 FINANCIAL DISCLOSURE AND CONFLICTS OF INTEREST

In "Financial Disclosure by Clinical Investigators" (21 *CFR* 54), the FDA states,

> [The] FDA may consider clinical studies inadequate and the data inadequate if, among other things, appropriate steps have not been taken in the design, conduct, reporting, and analysis of the studies to minimize bias. One potential source of bias in clinical studies is a financial interest of the clinical investigator in the outcome of the study because of the way payment is arranged (e.g., a royalty) or because the investigator has a proprietary interest in the product (e.g., a patent) or because the investigator has an equity interest in the sponsor of the covered study. This section and conforming regulations require an applicant whose submission relies in part on clinical data to disclose certain financial arrangements between sponsor(s) of the covered studies and the clinical investigators and certain interests of the clinical investigators in the product under study or in the sponsor of the covered studies. FDA will use this information, in conjunction with information about the design and purpose of the study, as well as information obtained through on-site inspections, in the agency's assessment of the reliability of the data.[33]

Requirements for Financial Disclosure

In the same guidance (21 *CFR* 54), the FDA states that it requires the following:

- Certification that no financial arrangements with an investigator have been made when the study outcome could affect compensation; that the investigator has no proprietary interest in the tested product; that the investigator does not have a significant equity interest in the sponsor of the covered study; and that the investigator has not received significant payments of other sorts; and/or
- Disclosure of specified financial arrangements and any steps taken to minimize the potential for bias.

Disclosable Financial Arrangements

The "financial arrangements" mentioned immediately above include the following:

- Compensation made to the investigator in which the value of compensation could be affected by the outcome of the study. This requirement applies to all covered studies ongoing or completed as of 2 February 1999.
- A proprietary interest in the tested product, including, but not limited to, a patent, trademark, copyright, or licensing agreement. This requirement applies to all covered studies ongoing or completed as of 2 February 1999.
- Any equity interest in the sponsor of a covered study, that is, any ownership interest, stock options, or other financial interest whose value cannot be readily determined through reference to public prices. This requirement applies to all covered studies, whether ongoing or completed.
- Any equity interest in a publicly held company that exceeds $50,000 in value. These must be disclosed only for covered clinical studies that are ongoing on or after 2 February 1999. The requirement applies to interests held during the time the clinical investigator is

carrying out the study and for one year following completion of the study.

- Significant payments of other sorts, which are payments with a cumulative monetary value of $25,000 or more, made by the sponsor of a covered study to the investigator or to the investigators' institution, to support activities of the investigator exclusive of the costs of conducting the clinical study or other clinical studies (for example, a grant to fund ongoing research, compensation in the form of equipment, or retainers paid for ongoing consultation or honoraria), during the time the clinical investigator is carrying out the study and for one year following completion of the study. This requirement applies to payments made on or after 2 February 1999.

Issues relating to financial disclosure can have an effect on human subjects and their decisions to participate in a clinical trial, as well as on the investigator, whose judgment may be affected by financial incentives or a preferred outcome for the study. Some centers inform subjects of the funding source for the clinical trial. Consider including a statement such as the following:

> The study sponsor is providing funds to the [study doctor or institution] on a per-patient basis for conducting this clinical trial. If you would like further details regarding the funding of this trial, please contact Institutional Review Board at [include phone number].

If it is determined that your institution or practice—or someone associated with the conduct of the study at your institution or your practice—has a disclosable financial conflict of interest, appropriate management of such conflict might include adding a statement to the consent form that addresses the conflict, for example:

> The principal investigator for this study has a significant financial interest that could be affected by the outcome of this study.

3.5 ASSENT IN CHILD SUBJECTS

Although children are not capable of giving legally valid consent, they may be able to *assent* or to *dissent* from participation. *Assent* is "knowledgeable agreement" to participate in a research study and should be used whenever the potential subject has sufficient capacity to understand what is happening and to express his or her wishes. The assent process requires that the investigator and the parent(s) discuss with the child what participation in the research study will involve as well as the possible risks and benefits. Federal regulations require that assent be obtained from all subjects who are capable of assenting unless certain conditions are met. When determining if minors are capable of giving assent, factors such as the age, maturity, psychological state, and medical condition of potential subjects must be considered. If the condition is life-threatening and the research presents the prospect of benefit, the IRB may vote that assent be waived.[34] Some organizations allow verbal assent while others require a written document.

A sample form is presented in Figure 3.5.[35] This form is most often used with younger children. Older teens may be able to assent using a consent form if it is appropriately written. Check the IRB's policy.

3.6 SAMPLE HIPAA AUTHORIZATION FORM

A separate form is necessary when the required privacy language of HIPAA is not incorporated within the body of the consent (see Figure 3.6).[36] The authorization form must include the following required elements in order to be in compliance with HIPAA legislation.

Pediatric Subject Assent Form

Project Title: ______________________________

Protocol Number: ______________________________

Investigator(s): ______________________________

Sponsor: ______________________________

We are doing a research study. A research study is a special way to find out about something. We are trying to find out how a special drug can be used to treat high blood pressure in children. You are being asked to be in this study because you have high blood pressure. Your blood pressure was measured using a blood pressure cuff at the doctor's office.

There will be about 210 children with high blood pressure in this study, some from the United States.

If you decide that you want to be in this study, you will come back to see the study doctor about 7 times over the next few months. If you are taking medicine for your high blood pressure, you will have to stop taking it. We will ask you to tell us how you feel, what medicines you are taking, and what problems you are having, if any.

We want to tell you about some of the things that might happen to you if you are in this study. The study doctor will give you a physical exam and measure your height and weight. This will not hurt. Your blood will be drawn with a needle about 2 times and that may hurt a little. You may get a small bruise or a sore where the needle went into your skin. We will look at your heartbeat with a special machine called an ECG twice; this will not hurt at all. We will take your blood pressure and heart rate at every visit. The blood pressure cuff will squeeze your arm and you may feel it as a pressure for a little while. We will count your heart rate to see how fast your heart is beating; this will not hurt. We will ask you to give us some of your urine in a cup about three times. If you are female and have started your menstrual periods, your urine will be tested to see if you are pregnant at the beginning of the study and at the end.

The study drug will be assigned by chance, like pulling numbers from a hat, to see which strength of study drug you will receive. During this study, you could receive 1 of 5 different strengths of the active study drug or you could receive a placebo tablet (a tablet that looks like the study drug, but does not have any of the medication the study drug has).

If you weigh less than 110 lbs., you will be randomly assigned to one of four treatment groups below:

- Placebo (no active medication)
- 2 mg of study drug
- 8 mg of study drug or
- 16 mg of study drug

[Continued on next page.]

Figure 3.5. Sample pediatric subject assent form.

If you weigh more than 110 lbs., you will be randomly assigned to one of the four treatment groups below:

- Placebo (no active medication)
- 4 mg of study drug
- 16 mg of study drug
- 32 mg of study drug

Eveyone who decides to enter this study will be on placebo (no active medication) for 1 week.

You should take the study drug whenever your parents (or guardian) tell you to take it. You will be asked to take the study drug once a day at about the same time for 5 weeks. The study drug may make you feel tired, dizzy, may give you a headache, runny nose, sore throat, a cough, make your stomach hurt, may make you feel like you have to throw up or make you throw up, may give you diarrhea (the runs), make your back or chest hurt, cause your arms, legs, hands, and feet to hurt or to puff out or you might have other problems. Be sure to tell your parent/guardian when or if you feel any of these things.

If you decide to be in this study, some good things might happen to you. Your blood pressure may not be high while you are taking the study drug. But we don't know for sure that these things will happen. There is a possibility that your blood pressure will not be lowered. Your blood pressure may not get better or may get worse if you are taking the placebo (no active medication) tablets. We might also find out things that will help other children some day.

There are definite risks to an unborn child if you were to become pregnant during the study. During pregnancy, this study drug can cause injury and even death to a developing unborn baby.

If you have started menstrual periods:

- **By signing this form, you confirm you are as sure as can be that you are not pregnant now and have no intention of becoming pregnant during this study.**
- **By signing this form, you agree that you will not have sex or if you do, you will use one of the following birth control methods: barrier method (sponge, diaphragm, or condom) plus spermicidal foam, oral (the "pill") or implanted contraceptives (Norplant).**
- **A urine pregnancy test will be done to confirm that you are not pregnant before you take part in this study as well as at the end of the study.**

Throughout the study, the study doctor or a member of the study staff will ask you about your menstrual period and the possibility of pregnancy. If they feel it is necessary, the study doctor or a member of the study staff can request additional pregnancy tests.

[Continued on next page.]

Figure 3.5, continued.

If at any time during this study you think you might be pregnant, or later learn that you were pregnant during the study, you must contact the study doctor immediately for further instructions. Your parent(s) or guardian(s) may have access to the pregnancy test results taken during this study.

Your parents (or guardian) must say it is okay for you to be in this study.

This study will not cost you or your parents (or guardian) any money.

You can ask the nurses and doctors questions any time.

You don't have to be in this study. We will tell you about the other things we can do for your high blood pressure.

When we are done with the study, we will write a report about what we found out. We won't use your name in the report.

You don't have to be in this study. It's up to you. If you say okay now, but you want to stop later, that's okay too. All you have to do is tell us.

If you want to be in this study, please sign your name. We will give you a copy of this form for you to keep.

I, ______________________________, want to be in this research study.
(Print your name here)

______________________________ (Sign your name here)	______________________________ Date of signature
______________________________ Signature of person obtaining this assent	______________________________ Date of signature
______________________________ Printed name of person obtaining this assent	
______________________________ Witness's* signature	______________________________ Date of signature
______________________________ Printed name of witness*	

* Witness is a 3rd party not related to the study or the subject

In addition to advising the above subject of other forms of treatment and therapy that are appropriate, I have offered an opportunity for further explanation of the risks and discomforts that are, or may be associated with this study, and to answer any further questions relating to it.

______________________________ Investigator's signature	______________________________ Date of signature

Figure 3.5, continued.

General Requirements

- The authorization must be written in plain language.
- A signed and dated copy of the authorization form must be given to the individual.

Core Elements

- A description of the information to be used or disclosed that identifies the information in a specific and meaningful fashion.
- Name or other specific identification of person(s) or a class of persons who are authorized to use or disclose the protected health information (PHI).
- Name or other specific identification of person(s) or a class of persons who are authorized to make the requested use or disclosure of the PHI.
- A description of each purpose of the requested use or disclosure. The statement "at the request of the individual" may be sufficient if the statement of purpose is not provided.
- An expiration date or expiration event. One may use "end of the research study" or none.
- The signature of the subject and the date the authorization was signed.

Required Statements

- A statement that subjects have the right to withdraw their authorization at any time; includes notification that such withdrawal must be in writing, and, if applicable, an explanation of the exceptions to the right to revoke.
- A statement informing subjects that once their PHI has been disclosed, it is possible that the receiver may redisclose the information. Subjects must know that at this point their personal information is no longer protected by federal privacy regulations.
- A statement that informs subjects that they may review and/or copy any PHI that is disclosed.
- A statement that tells subjects that they may refuse to sign the authorization and that choosing to refuse to sign the authorization will not affect their treatment.
- Subjects who were enrolled prior to 14 April 2003 do not have to be reconsented.
- Ongoing research projects will require an authorization form or consent modifications at the time of continuing review; however, if the consent form is not revised at any time after 14 April 2003, and subjects are not reconsented, it is possible that some subjects will not be required to sign an authorization.

Protected Health Information (PHI) Includes Any of the Following Items

- Name
- Social Security Number
- Geographic subdivision (that is, address and zip code)
- Medical record number
- All dates (that is, date of birth, admission date)
- Health plan number
- Telephone/fax number
- E-mail address
- Account number
- Vehicle identifier/serial number
- Certificate/license number
- Device identifier/serial number
- IP address
- URL
- DNA, tissue sample, or any other material that may contain identifiable characteristics
- Photo
- Biometric identifier

Authorization for Release of Health Information for Research Purposes

Principal Investigator: ____________________

Protocol #: ____________________

Sponsor: ____________________

Protocol Title: ____________________

The Health Insurance Portability & Accountability Act (HIPAA) is a federal law designed to protect the privacy of your health information. During your participation in this research study, your private health information will be used and additional information about you may be generated. The study doctor must get your permission before using or sharing any of your health information relating to this research study. This authorization form will explain what information will be obtained, how that information will be used and with whom it will be shared.

Private Health Information that will be used and disclosed includes:

- Your research records and supporting information from your medical records,
- Laboratory test results,
- Information obtained from the procedures used to determine your eligibility for the study and information obtained and observations made in the course of the study,
- Billing records, and
- Results from diagnostic and medical procedures including but not limited to x-rays, physical examinations, and medical history.

Your private health information will be used by the study doctor to conduct this research study and some of the information may be used in making decisions about your medical care. The study sponsor will use this information to analyze and make conclusions about the results of the study. Information about you will be reviewed when this study is monitored for quality assurance purposes. This information may also be used for additional research and development, regulatory and manufacturing activities, for reporting side-effects to the FDA and other government health agencies, and to support marketing claims about the study drug. The study results might also be published in medical journals. If the study results are published or used to support marketing claims, you will not be identified.

In addition to the study doctor and the sponsor, your private health information may also be used and shared with:

- The study staff and other representatives of the institution
- Individuals working for the sponsor
- Other companies owned by or associated with the sponsor or clinical research organization and the people working for these companies
- The Institutional Review Board
- The U.S. Food and Drug Administration and other government agencies
- Government agencies in other countries
- Accrediting agencies
- Data safety monitoring boards
- Health insurers/payors

Once your health information has been given by the study doctor to parties listed above who are not healthcare providers or otherwise subject to federal health privacy laws, U.S. federal privacy laws may no longer protect it. The information could be used or disclosed in ways other than those described in this authorization form. [Continued on next page.]

Figure 3.6. Sample HIPAA authorization form.

Authorization to Use and Disclose
By signing this authorization form, you are giving your study doctor permission to use and disclose your study information as described in this authorization form. You are also giving permission for review of your medical records by the parties listed above.

You do not have to sign this authorization. If you decide not to sign this authorization it will not affect your treatment. You will not lose any benefits or legal rights to which you are entitled. However, you will not be able to participate in the study.

Revoking Authorization
You may revoke (cancel) this authorization at any time by notifying the study doctor in writing [fill in name and address of PI here]. If you choose to revoke your authorization, the information that has already been collected cannot be withdrawn if it has been incorporated into the study data. Even if you withdraw your permission, Institution may keep, use, or disclose existing information needed for the integrity of the research, but will not collect any more information from you. Once you revoke your authorization you can no longer continue to participate in the study.

Access Information Collected
You will not be allowed to review the information collected during the course of the study until after the study is completed. When the study is over, you will have the right to access your information and you may request correction of any errors that you may find. To request this information, you may contact [fill in name of PI] at [fill in PI's phone number here].

Notice Concerning HIV-Related Information

If you are authorizing the release of HIV-related information, you should be aware that the recipient(s) is/are prohibited from redisclosing any HIV-related information without your authorization unless permitted to do so under federal or state law. You also have a right to request a list of people who may receive or use your HIV-related information without authorization. If you experience discrimination because of the release or disclosure of HIV-related information, you may contact your State Division of Human Rights at [fill in phone number here; also, add agencies and phone numbers appropriate for your state and institution here].

Expiration of Authorization
This authorization form will not expire. The information that is used and disclosed may continue to be used for many years.

You will receive a signed copy of this form.

________________________________ ____________________
Signature of subject | Date of signature

____
Printed name of subject

____
Signature of person obtaining this authorization

If signed by legally authorized representative:

________________________________ ____________________
Signature of legally authorized representative | Date of signature

________________________________ ____________________
Printed name of legally authorized representative | Relationship to subject

Figure 3.6, continued.

3.7 CONSENT FOR SUB-STUDIES

There may be pharmacogenetic studies or other types of sub-studies done in conjunction with the primary study. The same guidelines that apply to the standard informed consent document also apply to consent documents used for sub-studies. Additionally, the consent form must address the following:

- Is participation in the main study contingent upon participation in the sub-study?
- How long will the subject's samples be stored?
- If the subject decides to withdraw from the sub-study, will his or her sample be destroyed or returned?
- Will samples be stored for future use? If so, for what purpose? The IRB must also approve the future use of the samples.
- Is the sample identifiable or non-identifiable? There are risks associated with both. These risks must also be included in the consent form. It is possible that a commercial or marketable product may be developed as a result of the research done with a subject's sample. This is an area of the consent where you may encounter exculpatory language. The type of exculpatory statement to be avoided may be similar to the following: "You voluntarily donate your samples and you give up all claims to personal benefit from any commercial products that may be developed." Also, avoid language such as, "The sponsor will be the owner of any data or derivative materials generated from the study," as it may be construed as giving the sponsor property rights, thus waiving the rights of the subject.
- Instead, include a sentence such as,

  It is possible that the sponsor may develop a commercial product as a result of the data that is collected as part of this study, but there are no plans for you to profit financially from such a product should this occur.

3.8 SAMPLE CONSENT FORM FOR GENETIC TESTING AND/OR TISSUE BANKING[37]

A sample consent form is given in Figure 3.8.

3.9 SPONSORS' EFFORTS TO IMPROVE THE INFORMED CONSENT PROCESS

In a proactive effort, sponsors may go beyond providing individual templates for separate studies that are then edited by investigators to meet local IRB requirements; recently, some sponsors are partnering with IRBs to create "master consent form templates." IRBs may review and approve in advance sections of the consent form that consistently remain unchanged. This language, once approved, can be used in every consent form submitted by that sponsor. If these uniform elements are incorporated into the consent form, the approval process is faster and more efficient.

Often, sponsors ask to review any revisions that are made to their individual consent templates prior to and after IRB review. When this is the case, sponsors should keep in mind that IRBs adhere to strict submission deadlines, and it is important that sponsors return these consent documents as quickly as possible in order to avoid a delay of study start-up as a result of waiting for the next scheduled IRB meeting.

3.10 COMMON PROBLEMS WITH CONSENT FORM TEMPLATES RECEIVED FROM STUDY SPONSORS

- The document is written in technical terms and uses medical jargon.

Assent Form for Genetic Testing and/or Tissue Banking

Introduction
You are being asked to provide 1 additional blood sample (about X teaspoonfuls) for the study described below.

You do not have to agree to be in this additional study in order to be in the main study of Drug XX and Drug YY.

DNA is the material in your body's cells (genes) that passes on characteristics that are inherited from one generation to the next (like hair and eye color).

DNA will be extracted from your blood sample in a laboratory so that your genetic information can be used to study whether your response to treatment with Drug XX and any side-effects that you may have developed that are related to your genetic identity. This area of research is called "pharmacogenetics," because we are striving to understand how genes influences the different responses people have to the same drug. The goal of this research is to find variations in DNA that will help identify persons with [name of disease or condition] that will have the best response to Drug XX or to identify persons who will have fewer side-effects in order to maximize their benefit from Drug XX.

This is an experimental research study designed specifically to evaluate the relationship of your individual DNA to any improvement in your condition seen with Drug XX or to any side-effects that may arise during treatment. This research study is focused on studying the role genes play in [the disease or condition] and the responses of the subjects to Drug XX.

Scope of the Project
This study is being conducted at approximately XX research centers and is expected to involve about XX subjects.

Identified Samples [when applicable]
Your sample will be identified by your subject number, not your name. Only the investigator and the sponsor of the study will be able to link your subject number with your name. Neither you nor your doctor will be given the results of the testing [when applicable].

Non-Identified Samples [when applicable]
Your sample will be given a number that cannot be linked with you. Your sample will be stored with hundreds of other non-identified samples from [name of institution]. Neither you nor your doctor will be given the results of the testing.

Physical Risk—Blood Draws [when applicable]
Although the taking of the blood sample causes no serious problems for most people, it can cause some bleeding, bruising, tiredness, dizziness, and/or discomfort at the injection site.

Other Collection Procedures [when applicable]
[Describe procedure(s) and attendant risks.]

Physical Risk—Nonphysical Risk [when applicable]
There is a chance you may be the subject of discrimination if the results of the testing show a

[Continued on next page.]

Figure 3.8. Sample assent form for genetic testing and/or tissue banking.

genetic disorder. You might be denied a job or promotion, or denied health or life insurance if employers or insurance companies find out. You may experience other forms of discrimination. We will not release any information to anyone without your written permission. However, it is possible that genetic information may be revealed to others through legal means and may affect your ability to obtain insurance or get a job. In cases where parents and children are both tested, tests may reveal the possibility that the father is not the biological parent.

Potential Benefits of Genetic Testing
This study may improve our understanding of the role of genes in [name of disease]. Information learned about the gene may increase general knowledge, provide scientists with information about disease and/or eventually lead to improved treatment. There will be no direct benefit to you or your family from participating in this study.

Confidentiality
[For sample language and a discussion of this topic, see Element 9, page 32].

Whom to Contact with Questions about the Study
[For sample language and a discussion of this topic, see Element 11, page 34].

Subject Injury
[For sample language and a discussion of this topic, see Element 10, page 33].

Copy of Consent
[For sample language and a discussion of this topic, see Element 2, page 35].

Subject's Withdrawal from the Study
You are free to withdraw from this study at any time without giving up anything you might otherwise be entitled to. Withdrawal will not have any negative effect on your medical care or anything else. The investigator may also decide to end your participation in the study at any time. You may request that your sample and data relating to it be destroyed at any time, but this will only be possible if the sample and data can be identified.

Use and Storage of Samples
No tests other than those described in this form will be performed on your sample without your permission. Your sample will be destroyed at the end of the testing process, which is estimated to take approximately 20 years.

[Or, for storage of samples for general research purposes:]
In addition to the research outlined in this consent form, your stored sample may be used for general research purposes if you allow it. Please tell us which of the following you agree to (initial all that apply):

___ The sample may be used for any research project. You do not need to contact me if the sample is to be used for other research even if the sample can be identified with me.
___ Future studies can be completed without contacting me if all identifying information is removed so that the sample can't be linked to me.
___ I must be contacted prior to using my sample for future studies so that I can decide if I want my sample to be included in the study.
___ Under no circumstances may my sample be used for future studies.

[Continued on next page.]

Figure 3.8, continued.

Please tell us (by initialing the applicable line) whether you authorize the researchers to contact you in the future:

__ I authorize the researchers to contact me in the future for research purposes.

__ I do not authorize the researchers to contact me in the future for research purposes.

Storage of Cell Lines [when applicable]

The investigator may want to use your sample to make a cell line, which means that the cells from your sample would be treated in such a way that they may live and divide outside the body, be frozen for storage indefinitely, and be thawed in the future and used for future genetic research. There are no plans to share with you any financial profits that may result from this research.

Please tell us (by initialing the applicable line) whether you authorize the investigator to use your sample to make a cell line:

__ I consent to using my sample to make a cell line.

__ I do not consent to my sample being used for a cell line.

Statement of Consent

You have read this consent form and all of your questions have been answered to your satisfaction. You voluntarily consent to be a subject in this research study and to the procedures described in this form. You have been told that there are no plans to share with you any financial profits that may result from the use of your sample. Your are not waiving any legal rights by signing this form. You will receive a copy of this form for your records.

_______________________________ _______________

Signature of subject Date signed

____

Printed name of subject

_______________________________ _______________

Signature of the person obtaining consent Date signed

Figure 3.8, continued.

- Exculpatory language is used in the document.
- Sponsors may require subjects' initials, or witness's and/or investigator's signatures; this may be contradictory to the institution's policy.
- Unclear or understated compensation for injury language. The provision or lack of compensation that the investigational site or sponsor will provide in case of injury should be clearly stated.
- Including the inclusion and exclusion criteria from the protocol.

3.11 TAKE AWAY MESSAGES

- It is a challenge to prepare a comprehensive, easy to read, "not too technical" informed consent document.
- Informed consent is a vital part of the research study process.
- We must strive to make the informed consent process as effective as possible.

NOTES

1. *The Nuremberg Code,* "Permissible Medical Experiments," *Trials of War Criminals before the Nuernberg Military Tribunals under Control Council Law No. 10: Nuernberg, October 1946–April 1949* (Washington, D.C.: U.S. Government Printing Office, n.d., vol. 2): 181-2; *http://ohsrod.nih.gov/nuremberg.php3,* accessed 10 July 2002.

2. Department of Health, Education

and Welfare, *The Belmont Report* (Washington, D.C.: U.S. Government Printing Office, 1988, 201/778-80319 GPO 887-809); originally published in 44 *Federal Register* (18 April 1979), 23192-7; *http://ohrp.osophs.dhhs.gov/human subjects/guidance/belmont.htm*, accessed 10 July 2002.

3. World Medical Association, *The Declaration of Helsinki, http://www.wma.net/e/ethicsunit/helsinki.htm*, accessed 10 July 2004.

4. 21 *CFR* 50.25; 45 *CFR* 46.116.

5. Ibid.

6. HIPAA Final Rule, *http://www.hhs.gov/ocr/hipaa/finalreg.html*, accessed 25 October 2002.

7. 21 *CFR* 50.25; 45 *CFR* 46.116,(a),(1).

8. Ibid.

9. Biomedical Research Alliance of New York, *Standard Operating Procedures, Policy on: Informed Consent* (Great Neck, N.Y.: BRANY, Institute for Research Education, 2002).

10. Ibid.

11. See note 7 above.

12. Ibid.

13. See note 9 above.

14. See note 7 above.

15. Ibid.

16. See note 13 above.

17. 21 *CFR* 50.25; 45 *CFR* 46.116,(a),(3).

18. 21 *CFR* 50.25; 45 *CFR* 46.116,(a),(4).

19. 21 *CFR* 50.25; 45 *CFR* 46.116,(a),(5).

20. 21 *CFR* 50.25; 45 *CFR* 46.116,(a),(6).

21. See note 9 above.

22. Ibid.

23. 21 *CFR* 50.25; 45 *CFR* 46.116,(a),(7).

24. 21 *CFR* 50.25; 45 *CFR* 46.116,(a),(8).

25. See note 9 above.

26. 21 *CFR* 50.25; 45 *CFR* 46.116,(b),(1).

27. 21 *CFR* 50.25; 45 *CFR* 46.116,(b),(2).

28. 21 *CFR* 50.25; 45 *CFR* 46.116,(b),(3).

29. 21 *CFR* 50.25; 45 *CFR* 46.116,(b),(4).

30. 21 *CFR* 50.25; 45 *CFR* 46.116,(b),(5).

31. 21 *CFR* 50.25; 45 *CFR* 46.116,(b),(6).

32. OPRR, Exculpatory *Language in Informed Consent Documents*, 15 November 1996, *http://ohrp.osophs.dhhs.gov/humansubjects/guidance/exculp.html*, accessed 9 July 2002.

33. 21 *CFR* 54.

34. 45 *CFR* 46.408A.

35. See note 9 above.

36. HIPAA Authorization form, *http://www.karenzupko.com/Communities/Ortho/HIPAAAuthorization Form Sample.doc*, accessed 20 October 2002; *Human Research Compliance Insider* (New York: Brownstone Publishers, November 2002).

37. See note 9 above.

4

The Trial Has Been Approved . . . What's Next?

Raffaella Hart, CIP

Chapter 4 will emphasize communication with the IRB after a clinical research project receives initial IRB approval. Because so many groups have an interest in any given clinical trial, it may be difficult to navigate the channels of communication in a way that best helps to protect human subjects.

This chapter will highlight the critical importance of ongoing IRB-investigator-sponsor communication that protects human subjects by considering the following topics:

4.1 Essential Communication
4.2 Your Project Is Approved . . . Now What?
4.3 Adverse Events
4.4 Data Safety Monitoring Boards and IRBs
4.5 Deviations from the Protocol
4.6 Continuing Review
4.7 Take Away Messages

4.1 ESSENTIAL COMMUNICATION

The IRB, investigators, and sponsors are the parties directly responsible for protecting human research subjects. These three groups should maintain frequent interaction, not only at a research project's initiation, but also for its duration. This is critically important to the safety of the research participants and to the validity and integrity of the data.

Investigators play a crucial role in interactions between IRBs and sponsors. Direct communication between IRBs and sponsors is less common, and sometimes is discouraged. Rather, investigators serve as principal intermediaries between IRBs and sponsors. Investigators, who are best-suited to facilitate the exchange of information, should be the individuals who are most familiar with sponsors' and IRBs' policies and procedures. When questions or concerns arise during the initial review of a research project, IRBs direct these questions to investigators, who can subsequently solicit additional information from sponsors, if necessary.

It is important to note that direct communication between sponsors and IRBs is a practice that has become more common with the advent of centralized and independent IRBs. Establishing a successful relationship and an avenue for communication between investigators, IRBs, and sponsors helps to ensure the protection of human subjects. This helps to keep everyone apprised of new information as it arises. Specifically, the reporting of any adverse event (AE) requires appropriate communication to help ensure the safety of subjects and the effective circulation of any new information. Such communication is essential and should occur throughout the life of a research project.

4.2 THE PROJECT IS APPROVED . . . NOW WHAT?

Once a clinical research project has earned approval by an IRB, various interactions take place between the investigator, the sponsor, and the IRB before the trial can start. The investigator must ensure that the IRB-approved informed consent document is available and that the study supplies are complete and readily accessible once the trial is initiated. For industry-sponsored trials, it is important for the investigator to develop a relationship with the monitor, or clinical research associate, who has been designated by the sponsor for the project. The monitor will serve as the sponsor's primary liaison with the investigational site, and will be a vital resource for the investigator.

Understanding the Process of Informed Consent

Central to the success of a clinical trial is the ability to properly obtain informed consent. To do this, the investigator and members of the research staff must be familiar with the consent document. In industry-sponsored research, the sponsor often sends a template for the informed consent document to the site. Nevertheless, it is imperative that the investigator be involved in all aspects of preparing the consent document, and review the IRB-approved version to ensure that all of the necessary elements are present. It is even more important for the investigator to ensure that the document presents information to research participants in a clear, practical, and complete manner. The investigator should refer to the IRB's and/or sponsor's policies, as well as any regulations that pertain to consent (and assent, if applicable); if appropriate, the consent document should be revised as necessary before the study begins.

Know the IRB's Standard Operating Procedures

Once the trial has been approved, the investigator must ensure access to, and be familiar with, the procedures of the IRB of record and maintain a copy of these standard operating procedures (SOPs) in the study file.[1] It is here that study staff will learn the specific procedures to follow, as well as obtain the forms necessary to submit amendments and AE reports to the IRB. The investigator must be aware of all reporting requirements, including those dictated by the IRB, the sponsor, and the applicable federal and state authorities. Knowledge of this information helps prevent delays in processing of amendments, and thus the initiation and conduct of the study.

Using the IRB's Submission Forms

An IRB usually requires completion of specific forms to facilitate the review of amendments and AEs. These forms prompt the investigator to include all necessary components of the amendment or AE, and to make a determination about whether other aspects of the clinical trial must be modified. Specific forms are preferable to a letter from the sponsor or the investigator describing the submission. For example, when an investigator writes a letter to an IRB requesting review of an item, he or she may fail to indicate whether the informed consent document needs to be revised as a result. Similarly, an investigator may omit required supporting documentation, such as a summary of protocol revisions or a copy of a safety update, that require modification to the consent form. IRB submission forms help to remind investigators about how to follow the IRB's procedures, and help to provide consistency in the reporting of AEs and in the review of amendments.

Amendments

Amendments, or changes in previously approved research, require IRB approval before they may be implemented. As a rule of thumb, *amendments* can be defined as a modification to the research project as previously approved by the IRB. Amendments might include, but are not limited to, modification of protocol procedures, change in the study's duration, updates to the investigator's brochure for the study agent, addition or substitution of investigators and sub-investigators, modification of or foreign language translation of the informed consent document, advertisements, and administrative revisions. The IRB will determine whether the submitted amendments may add risk to subjects and whether the amendments are subject to expedited review or require review by the convened committee. Federal regulations describe types of "minor changes" that may be reviewed by the IRB via the mechanism of expedited review.[2] The types of IRB review were discussed in more detail in chapter 2.

4.3 ADVERSE EVENTS

Definitions of an *adverse event* vary across the different regulatory agencies that govern clinical trials. "The notification requirements described in the Common Rule [45 *CFR* 46] define AEs as 'unanticipated problems' involving risks to study participants or others. Generally, the [sponsors] establish operational definitions of AEs that apply to the particular trial."[3] The U.S. Food and Drug Administration (FDA), in 21 *CFR* Part 312, defines AEs as "any untoward medical occurrence that may present itself during treatment or administration with a pharmaceutical product, and which may or may not have a causal relationship with the treatment."[4] In the guideline "Clinical Safety Data Management: Definitions and Standards for Expedited Reporting," the FDA further clarifies and defines a serious AE that stems from a drug study as:

- Any untoward medical occurrence that at any dose results in death,
- Is life-threatening,
- Requires inpatient hospitalization or prolongation of existing hospitalization,
- Creates persistent or significant disability/incapacity, or congenital anomaly/birth defects.[5]

Many sponsors and IRBs rely on this definition, as it offers a more conservative approach to classifying AEs, and provides a more global approach to making an assessment. This conservative approach adds to the burden of IRBs and investigators, as it often calls for more frequent reporting and reviewing of AE reports.

The interpretation of what constitutes an AE can be somewhat imprecise and is left, to some degree, to the investigator, which can affect the consistency of AE reporting. Researchers who report AEs are asked to report on the event's level of seriousness and expectedness, degree of relationship to the study agent, and whether the event was resolved. In making this assessment, the investigator must take into account the known characteristics of the underlying disease or the indication under study, and then determine whether the AE is associated with the use of the investigational agent. Inconsistencies in reporting by different investigators may result in unbalanced information for the same AE, contributing to a lack of consistency in determining the relationship between the AE and the research.

Reporting AEs—What Is an IRB's Barometer?

It is up to the IRB to determine which AEs will be reported at an investigational site. Practically, however, sponsors may also play a role by requiring the reporting of AEs that may fall outside an IRB's reporting criteria. Investigators are responsible for reporting all serious adverse events (SAEs) that occur at their site to the IRB and to the research sponsor. The sponsor then disseminates this information—often called IND (investigational new drug) safety reports[6] or "Dear Doctor letters"—to other sites that are involved in a research study that uses the same study agent. The IRBs at the other sites will then review the reports. Specific IRB reporting requirements may vary, and investigators should be aware of the policies at their own organization.

In large, multi-center research projects, hundreds of AE reports pertaining to the agents under study may be generated and disseminated to all investigational sites. These reports are often referred to as IND (investigational new drug) Safety Reports, and are produced in various formats, according to the sponsor's practice. MedWatch is the FDA safety information and AE reporting program.[7] Many clinical research sponsors utilize the MedWatch reporting form, which allows more uniform review of new safety information pertaining to medical products. Regardless of the format, it is important to make certain that, at a minimum, these vital elements of the AE are described in the report:

- Description and brief history of the research subject,
- When and where the AE occurred,
- Whether this is an initial or follow-up report,
- Whether the investigator and/or sponsor believe there is any relationship of the event to the study agent.

Again, it is important for the investigator and the IRB to consider whether or not the informed consent document should be revised to incorporate the new safety information that is contained within the AE report.

It would be helpful to standardize the reporting process, so that everyone would follow the same convention, obtain the same safety information, and apply it the same way. Unfortunately this is not the case, and the result is that sponsors, investigators, and IRBs find it difficult to derive meaningful information from these reports. Even the guidance from the National Institutes of Health (NIH) on reporting AEs to IRBs describes how AE reporting has become one of the most "burdensome and confusing" aspects of conducting clinical trials, largely due to the different regulations that have been issued by NIH and FDA.[8] Further complicating the issue, IRBs set their own parameters for AE reporting, which can confuse sponsors and investigators in determining what events are reportable; in multi-center studies, there may be many local IRBs involved, each using its own AE reporting structure.[9]

Reporting AEs— A Necessary "Burden"

Whatever definition is used, it is important to remember that "untoward" and/or "unexpected" events must be communicated through the proper channels, and that the outcome of this information is that pertinent new information is effectively communicated to research participants when necessary. Human subjects should be informed of any new information that may affect their willingness to continue participating in research. While ongoing communication among IRBs, sponsors, and investigators may not remedy the difficulties encountered in extracting meaningful information from AE reports, the regular interaction of these groups will help to ensure that, even if it is done in a somewhat "burdensome and confusing" manner, the information is exchanged,[10] and we are taking steps toward ensuring protection of human subjects.

What Do IRBs Do with all the AE Reports?—The Role of the IRB in Interpreting AEs

IRBs must evaluate the information generated and use it to take the appropriate actions to protect human subjects. What are these appropriate actions?

IRB review of AE reports generally falls into two categories: (1) reports of serious AEs that occur at an investigational site under the IRB's purview, and (2) IND safety reports, or reports of AEs that occur at other research sites using the same investigational agent. While safety reports provide information that is directly related to what is happening at the local research site, IND safety reports provide more generalizable, aggregate information related to the global use of the study agent.

If the relationship of an AE to the research is unclear, an IRB should request further details to help assess the impact on subjects' safety. Based on the severity of the AE and the event's impact on subjects' safety, an IRB may suspend or terminate its approval for a research project, require revision to the informed consent document or research protocol, or request additional information to address any concerns it may have. If a significant number of AEs are reported in a multi-center research project, but the relationship to the study agent is unclear, the IRB may request that the sponsor of the research develop a more formalized mechanism to monitor and analyze this information to more clearly evaluate the information and its potential impact on study subjects. A data and safety monitoring board, or DSMB, may perform this monitoring. DSMBs will be discussed in further detail later in this chapter.

Should This AE Be Submitted to the IRB?

IRBs are always being asked by investigators and sponsors, "Should this AE report be submitted to the IRB for review?" The answer is often unclear. If the answer is uncertain, the best course is to report the AE to the IRB to ensure that potentially important new information is not overlooked. Information pertaining to the frequency and nature of the AE in a given study population should be provided to the IRB, when it is available.

Other AEs: Non-Therapeutic, Observational, and Device Trials

What about the reporting of AEs in non-therapeutic studies and/or observational trials? Investigators should remember that different types of clinical research may result in different types of AEs. Risks and AEs that arise during a clinical research study may not always be physical in nature. A study may involve a survey or questionnaire that has the potential to distress subjects, or it may involve social or behavioral research, in which AEs might also be measured as changes in individual or social behavior. For example, in a study of a new drug to treat schizophrenia, an AE was reported in which the subject was arrested for theft. While the subject exhibited no abnormal physiological symptoms, the investigator deemed this event reportable and associated with the use of the study agent and/or the subject's condition.

AEs in Investigational Device Studies

In the studies of investigational medical devices, investigators are asked to report AEs experienced by subjects in the same way they would for the study of an investigational new drug, but the device manufacturers, importers, and user facilities are asked to report significant medical device AEs directly to the FDA using the Medical Device Reporting (MDR) System, so that AEs can be detected and corrected promptly.[11] The FDA's Center for Devices and Radiological Health provides further guidance for medical device reporting, available at *http://www.fda.gov/cdrh/mdr/mdr-general.html.*

When should AEs be reported? The FDA regulation states, "An investigator shall promptly report to the sponsor any adverse effect that may reasonably be regarded as caused by, or probably caused by, the drug. If the adverse effect is alarming, the investigator shall report the adverse effect immediately."[12] Similarly, an IRB generally describes its requirements, defines deadlines for reporting AEs, and provides the appropriate reporting mechanism. For example, an IRB may require that the initial report be submitted within 24 hours of the event's occurrence, followed by a written report in a defined number of days.

According to the International Conference on Harmonisation (ICH) Good Clinical Practice Guidelines (GPG), "All serious adverse events (SAE) should be reported immediately to the sponsor. . . . The immediate reports should be followed promptly by detailed, written reports. . . . The investigator should also comply with the applicable regulatory requirement(s) related to the reporting of unexpected SAE to the regulatory authorities and the IRB/IEC [independent ethics committee]."[13] In the interest of effectively protecting human subjects, the investigator and study staff should become familiar with all of the AE reporting requirements to which they are subject before a clinical trial begins.

4.4 DATA SAFETY MONITORING BOARDS AND IRBs

Data and safety monitoring boards (DSMBs) are independent bodies established to assess and anticipate developing safety issues indicated by the data collected throughout the life of a study. Because DSMBs usually have access to unblinded information, they may provide analysis of safety information in a more useful format; they can offer an analysis of data collected across several investigational sites, and they can generate information about the outcomes of this data, and may identify new safety concerns, if and when they arise. IRBs should not function as DSMBs, but should ensure that the appropriate mechanisms are in place to monitor data collection to ensure subjects' safety in a clinical research project.[14] As the NIH guidance notes, "The DSMB monitoring function is above and beyond the oversight traditionally provided by IRBs and as such is particularly important for multi-center trials."[15]

IRB members may have difficulty assessing the relevance of an isolated AE report without information pertaining to the total number of subjects in the study who may have experienced the same AE, compared with how many subjects are currently enrolled in the study. For example, if an IND safety report indicates an unexpected occurrence of "gastrointestinal bleed," an IRB can better assess the report if it has information about the frequency of the event at all sites using the study agent. This is where the DSMB comes in. This type of information is often best provided by interim reports from a DSMB that has been established for that particular trial, or for the agent under study. For research sponsored by the NIH, DSMBs are required to provide IRBs with copies of these reports. Although it is not required, other research sponsors often employ the same practice, and many IRBs require these reports regardless of sponsorship.

NIH guidance addresses the "need for communication between the DSMB and IRB."[16] The IRB can evaluate whether there is adequate monitoring of the safety of research subjects once a DSMB is established. The IRB can also evaluate the DSMB's monitoring plan and request modifications if the plan is deemed unsatisfactory.[17] The sponsor also has an obligation to transmit the DSMB report(s) to investigators in a timely and efficient manner. The investigators, in turn, are obligated to transmit the DSMB report(s) to the local IRB. The IRB may then suspend or terminate approval when an unexpected AE happens at its own site, or when it learns of an unexpected AE occurring at another investigational site. As the NIH guidance states, the IRB has authority to request DSMB reports and can make "reporting [of a summary of safety information] contingent on IRB approval for specific studies that are deemed appropriate. . . . An IRB should communicate concerns to the DSMB and/or [sponsor] if it believes that the safety of study participants is in jeopardy."[18]

DSMBs often schedule analysis of study data at various points throughout a study, but an IRB can prompt a DSMB to review study data at other necessary times. For example, consider an ongoing, multi-center clinical research study of subjects with sepsis, during which the investigator notices that subjects' clotting indices are increasing beyond expected levels. The investigator reports this information to the IRB, and the IRB suspends the research, pending a report from the sponsor and the DSMB. The DSMB's investigation reveals that the solution used to dilute the study agent contains a substance that affects laboratory results without posing harm to subjects. The study can be modified accordingly, if necessary, and can then continue.

4.5 DEVIATIONS FROM THE PROTOCOL

"Assurance of IRB Review," 21 *CFR* 321.66, a federal regulation, states, "The investigator shall also assure that he or she will promptly report to the IRB all changes in the research activity and all unanticipated problems involving risk to human subjects or others, and that he or she will not make any changes in the research without IRB approval, except where necessary to eliminate apparent immediate hazards to human subjects."[19] Form FDA 1572, "Statement of Investigator," includes a similar statement.[20] Investigators are required to sign this form for research projects that involve an IND or biologic agent. If investigators do not comply with this requirement, they may suffer serious repercussions; the FDA may limit their ability to perform research, or it may suspend or debar them.

What Constitutes a Deviation from the Protocol and Is the Deviation Reportable?

To maintain the integrity of the data collected, investigators should be encouraged to report all deviations from the protocol to the sponsor and to the IRB. In this way, the sponsor may make a determination about whether the data collected for the "deviated" subject will be valid in later data analyses, and the IRB may evaluate the deviation with respect to subjects' safety.

Defining Protocol Deviations

How can a deviation from the protocol be defined? Are deviations limited to "unanticipated problems involving risks to human subjects or others"? *Any procedure that is not prescribed by the protocol or the regulations governing the study may be considered a deviation.* Investigators may have difficulty conforming to some protocol requirements. However, investigators are responsible for carefully evaluating the protocol at the onset of the research project to ensure that they are able to meet the protocol's requirements.

Alternatively, the standard of care for a given procedure might change during the course of a study, and the investigator may need to modify the protocol for the benefit of subjects. For example: during a study of subjects with cancer, enough clinical evidence is gathered to support that the dose of radiation given to such patients as part of standard care should be increased for effectiveness, and the new dose has been put into practice universally. The protocol, however, prescribes a lower dose. In this scenario, the investigator, in the interest of providing the most effective care to study subjects, should request a modification of the protocol, obtain sponsor and IRB approval, and subsequently alter the radiation given to subjects.

Changes to and deviations from the protocol are generally unplanned. The investigator must promptly report such instances to the IRB and the sponsor. It is the IRB's responsibility to evaluate these instances, paying special attention to the impact on subjects' rights and safety. The sponsor will assess these issues as well as consider the validity of the trial data.

4.6 CONTINUING REVIEW

Substantive continuing review of ongoing clinical research projects is crucial to ensure the most effective protection of human subjects. It is the investigator's responsibility to ensure that the status of a research project is reported to the IRB prior to the expiration of the IRB's approval, and to do so with ample time to allow the IRB to review the investigator's application for renewal of the approval. Department of Health and Human Services (DHHS) regulations state, "an IRB shall conduct continuing review covered by this policy at intervals appropriate to the degree of risk, but not less than once per year. . . ."[21] For research that does not qualify for expedited review or that is not in an exempt category, the continuing review must take place by the convened IRB, and the review "must be substantive and meaningful."[22]

While regulations describe the minimum interval for performing continuing review, it is important that the investigator be aware of the local IRB's requirements, as they may call for more frequent review than those outlined in the regulations. IRBs need to ensure the protection of human subjects, and so may impose more stringent requirements for continuing review, depending on the research project's degree of risk. The regulations also give the IRB the authority to observe the informed consent and research processes so that it may assess whether the rights and welfare of study subjects are being adequately protected, or protected at all.[23]

To give the IRB an adequate "snapshot" of the clinical research project at the time of continuing review, investigators should include the following materials (at a minimum) with submissions for continuing approval.

Continuing Review Submissions Checklist

- Describe the current status of the research project. Is the study open to the entry of new subjects, or is it limited only to the follow up of subjects who have already enrolled?
- Indicate the status of all subjects involved in the clinical research project, including reasons for any withdrawals or screen failures.
- Provide the current, IRB-approved version(s) of the informed consent document(s), including foreign language translations, if applicable. This helps

the IRB ensure that the investigational site is using the appropriate version of the informed consent document.

- Provide any other subject-related literature (for example, questionnaires, subject diaries, dosing schedules, et cetera).
- Indicate whether any SAEs have occurred at your investigational site, and, if so, describe the relationship to the study agent. If the AEs have already been submitted to the IRB for review, provide a summary.
- Supply a report from the DSMB, or the most current safety monitoring information available to you. If the information is not available, indicate the reason(s) why.
- Furnish any recent literature about the study agent or the clinical research project that has yielded any new safety information.
- Summarize all protocol/study design modifications and informed consent document modifications, and indicate the status of their IRB approval.
- Note any additional training in good clinical research practice that has been completed by the investigator.
- Describe any changes to the status of potential conflicts of interest that may apply to the investigator or members of his/her immediate family (for example, outside interests, outside activities, gifts, gratuities, and entertainment from study sponsors or their competitors). Conflicts of interest are described in further detail in chapters 5 and 8.
- Note any changes in investigational site staff (for example, Form FDA 1572, subinvestigators, clinical research coordinators).

I Forgot to Submit My Continuing Review Form . . . What Now?

What are the implications of failing to report to the IRB? What happens if the continuing review does not take place before the expiration of IRB approval?[24] According to the applicable regulations, the IRB has the authority to suspend or terminate its approval. The IRB is also obligated to report significant lapses in IRB approval to FDA and/or the Office for Human Research Protections (OHRP), but FDA guidance suggests that the IRB need not report suspensions of a few days that are caused by failure to submit the appropriate documentation for re-approval prior to the expiration date.[25] The sponsor and/or regulatory authorities may also suspend the research in the interest of protecting human subjects and maintaining data integrity.[26]

What role is the IRB to play in monitoring, warning, and notifying investigators of upcoming expirations? It is the investigator's responsibility to ensure that the research proposal undergoes timely and continuing review. As a courtesy, most IRBs will remind investigators of continuing review deadlines. However, if a warning is not received, the investigator should maintain the responsibility of submitting continuing review in a timely manner.

4.7 TAKE AWAY MESSAGES

- Communication and interaction between the IRB, the investigator, and the sponsor is vital to effectively protect human subjects and to a safe and successful clinical research trial.
- Communication between the IRB, investigators, and sponsors should occur throughout the duration of a clinical research project.
- Investigators have the ultimate responsibility for communicating with IRBs.
- Investigators should be involved in all aspects of preparing consent documents and in the informed consent process.
- Know and follow your IRB's SOPs.
- Consider whether amendments and/or AEs will require modification of the consent form.

- Reporting requirements for AEs may differ. Make sure you know your IRB's reporting requirements.
- Although it is not desirable, protocol deviations may happen. Report them promptly to the IRB.
- Avoid a lapse in IRB approval and suspension of research. Avoid waiting until the last minute to submit continuing review applications.
- IRBs are not DSMBs, but IRBs use information supplied by DSMBs in their decision making.

NOTES

1. NIH, Notice 99-107, "Guidance on Reporting Adverse Events to Institutional Review Boards for NIH-Supported Multicenter Clinical Trials," release date 11 June 1999, *http://grants2.nih.gov/grants/guide/notice-files/not99-107. html*, accessed 6 June 2002.
2. 45 *CFR* 46.110; 21 *CFR* 56.110.
3. 21 *CFR*, "Chapter 1—Food and Drug Administration, DHHS; Part 312—Investigational New Drug Application," updated 1 April 2002, *http://www.access.gpo.gov/nara/cfr/*, accessed 6 June 2002. .
4. *CFR* 312, "Chapter 1—Food and Drug Administration, DHHS; Part 312—Investigational New Drug Application," updated 1 April 2002, *http://www.access.gpo.gov/nara/cfr/*, accessed 6 June 2002.
5. FDA, Center for Drug Evaluation and Research, "Guideline for Industry—Structure and Content of Clinical Study Reports," *Federal Register*, 17 July 1995, *http://www.fda.gov/cder/guidance/iche3.pdf*, accessed 6 June 2002.
6. See note 3 above.
7. 45 *CFR*, "Department of Health and Human Services; Part 46—Protection of Human Subjects; updated 1 October 2001," accessed 6 June 2002, *http://www.access.gpo.gov/nara/cfr/*.
8. See note 1 above.
9. See note 6 above.
10. Ibid.
11. FDA—Center for Devices and Radiological Health, "Reporting Problems With Medical Devices," *http://www.fda.gov/cdrh/mdr. html*, accessed 6 June 2002.
12. 21 *CFR* 312, "Chapter 1—Food and Drug Administration, DHHS; Part 312. 64(b)—Investigational New Drug application," updated 1 April 2002, *http://www.access.gpo.gov/nara/cfr/*, accessed 6 June 2002.
13. ICH Harmonized Tripartite Guideline, "Guideline for Good Clinical Practice E6," (recommended for adoption on 1 May 1996 by the ICH Steering Committee), *http://www.ich.org/pdfICH/e6.pdf*, accessed 6 June 2002.
14. E.A. Bankert and R.J. Amdur, "The IRB is not a data and safety monitoring board," *IRB: A Review of Human Subjects Research* 22, no. 6 (2000): 9-11.
15. See note 1 above.
16. Ibid.
17. Ibid.
18. Ibid.
19. 21 *CFR* 312.66.
20. 21 *CFR* 312, "Statement of Investigator," Form FDA 1572 (8/01).
21. 45 *CFR* 46.109(e).
22. OHRP, DHHS, "Guidance on Continuing Review," updated 11 July 2002, *http://ohrp.osophs.dhhs.gov/human subjects/guidance/contrev2002.html*, accessed 12 July 2002.
23. 45 *CFR* 46.109(e).
24. 45 *CFR* 46.113; 21 *CFR* 56.113.
25. See note 22 above.
26. 21 CFR 50 Subpart B; 45 CFR 46.101(a)(2). 21 *CFR*, "Volume 1—Food and Drug Administration, DHHS; Part 50—Protection of Human Subjects; Subpart B—Informed Consent of Human Subjects," updated 1 April 2003, *http://www. access data.fda.gov/scripts/cdrh/cfdocs/cfdocs/cfcfr/CFRSearch.dfm?CFRPart=50*, accessed 10 October 2003.

5

Financial Considerations and Their Impact on Human Subjects Protection

Eileen Hilton, MD

This chapter will address how financial issues in clinical research may affect the protection of human subjects. It will include the following discussions:

5.1 How Expensive Is It to Properly Staff and Run a Human Subjects Protections Program?
5.2 Charging for IRB Review
5.3 Financial Conflicts of Interest
5.4 Take Away Messages

5.1 HOW EXPENSIVE IS IT TO PROPERLY STAFF AND RUN A HUMAN SUBJECTS PROTECTIONS PROGRAM?

Several high-profile research trials, some involving gene therapy, have increased public concern about the welfare of human subjects in research.[1] Federal regulatory agencies have responded with an increase in oversight and compliance efforts. As a consequence, IRBs are faced with mounting workloads and staff shortages.

Since June 1998, the Office for Human Research Protections (OHRP, formerly the Office for Protection from Research Risk—OPRR) has conducted on-site reviews at several institutions. This represents a substantial increase from the previous year, when only one on-site inspection was performed.[2] These inspections have resulted in several well-publicized research suspensions at respected institutions.[3] The repercussions from these actions have reverberated throughout the academic and research community.

IRBs and officials at other research institutions sat up and took notice. The realization that suspensions can happen anywhere has increased self-examination of the systems and internal resources needed to comply with the requirements for conducting quality and ethical human research. These federal investigations have had positive effects. IRBs have developed educational programs for investigators, administrators, and IRB members; created tracking systems for audits and the reporting of adverse events (AEs); and enlisted staff to ensure investigator and institutional compliance in human subject protections.

As a by-product, the volume of paperwork that IRBs face has increased enormously. There is an ever-increasing amount of material submitted to IRBs for review and written response. It is sometimes difficult to separate the important matters that are relevant to human subject protections from *pro forma* submissions sent for other reasons. Additionally, more protocols are being reviewed by IRBs because the number of clinical trials being performed has increased. Additional personnel are needed to assist overburdened staff.

How many employees does an organization require to support an IRB's administrative functions? There are few guidelines to help determine the optimal number of IRB staff necessary to perform all of the requisite tasks. In the past, an individual IRB coordinator may have managed several hundred protocols per year. Many would now agree that this is not feasible, as the volume of adverse event and investigational new drug (IND) safety reports has increased dramatically. Other work has also increased, as IRB coordinators are now occupied with the education of investigators and IRB members, as well as the additional responsibility of collecting and monitoring information regarding conflicts of interest.

So how does an administration determine how many employees are needed? Many organizations use a calculation of the number of actions processed as a gauge of how many staff should be assigned. Additionally, workload distribution may be changed to process the enormous number of requests submitted to the IRB. In the past, an individual IRB coordinator may have done it all—scheduled meetings, organized agendas, readied new submissions, and managed AE reporting and a myriad other tasks. Now, larger organizations may distribute tasks differently. For example, one individual may be solely delegated to handling AE reports, another to expedited review, and a third to managing compliance and policy issues.

What Other Factors Contribute to the Increasing Cost of Maintaining a Compliant Human Research Protections Program?

Education

In 2000, both the National Institutes of Health (NIH) and the U.S. Public Health Service (PHS) issued new policies on educating IRBs and researchers. The PHS guidelines expand on the NIH's guidelines in the following ways. Instruction must be given in (1) data acquisition, management, sharing, and ownership; (2) mentor/trainee responsibilities; (3) publication practices and responsible authorship; (4) peer review; (5) collaborative science; (6) human subjects; (7) research involving animals; (8) research misconduct; (9) conflict of interest and commitment; and (10) compliance with existing PHS and institutional policies.[4]

Meeting these new educational requirements has added additional costs for institutions. Many institutions hired educators, and others employed subcontractors from outside educational organizations. This educational training is essential, as it informs all clinical coordinators, investigators, IRB staff, and IRB members of federal regulations regarding human subject protections. As human subject protections requirements change frequently, education, as an ongoing process, is costly. More detailed information on education is presented in chapter 6.

Compliance

Some IRBs have expanded their staff to include internal auditors or monitors. In the 1998 report from the U.S. Office of the Inspector General (OIG), a consistent finding was the superficiality of continuing IRB review.[5] OIG reported that reviews were limited to paperwork submitted by researchers. They noted the lack of on-site audits or monitoring. While there are no clear-cut regulations on the number or selection of ongoing and past trials that should be audited, it is clear that the federal government would like to see more on-site monitoring by institutions to assure human subjects protections. This too results in a significant increase in expense for IRBs.

Gene Therapy

A great deal of publicity has surrounded gene therapy research at a few academic institutions.[6] The alleged failure in oversight by the institutions during these trials has prompted some institutions to add internal "gene therapy" monitors to the payroll. This is in addition to the institutional biosafety committees already in place. These positions require an individual who has considerable clinical and regulatory expertise.

Who Will Bear the Burden of All of This Additional Expenditure to Ensure the Protection of Human Subjects?

Is this solely an institutional responsibility, or should the sponsors of the research share the expense? Support for IRB functions has traditionally been provided by the institutional overhead charged to NIH and to industry sponsors. It is not clear that these resources will continue to be sufficient to cover the costs of protecting human subjects. Hence, institutions are looking for additional outside support for these essential functions.

5.2 CHARGING FOR IRB REVIEW

In the past, charging for IRB review was rare in academic institutions. IRBs were staffed with a few administrators and their workload was manageable. Institutional costs were reasonable, and the revenue accrued from institutional overhead was sufficient to cover the expense of an IRB. This has changed for all of the reasons previously cited. Increasingly, organizations have realized the need to share the costs and responsibilities of human subject protections. Many charge for initial review only—with fees ranging from $500 to $2,000. This may change as the number of AE and safety reports increase. Most sponsors realize that the burden must be shared and incorporate these IRB costs into their clinical trial budgets. NIH has also recognized the need for additional support, and, in 2002, awarded grants in support of improving IRB performance in federally funded institutions.

How Do IRBs Actually Collect these Charges?

This can be challenging. Some IRBs require "up front" payment from investigators or sponsors before they will review the project. In some cases investigator research funds are debited when proceeds are submitted. Others invoice sponsors and/or investigators. This is more expensive, as it requires staff to follow up on unpaid fees.

What about Fees Charged by IRBs for Research that Is Federally Funded or Initiated by an Investigator?

In general, IRBs do not charge for review of federally funded research, as the institutional overhead negotiated with the government is supposed to include support of IRB functions.

5.3 FINANCIAL CONFLICTS OF INTEREST

The following is a discussion of financial conflicts of interest for researchers and institutions. Chapter 8 addresses conflicts of interest for IRB members.

When his son, Jesse Gelsinger, died after participating in a gene transfer trial, Paul Gelsinger directed these comments to researchers: "Approach the protection of human research subjects the same as you would your own children and with the same intent that Jesse had and you will have it right . . . not for recognition or for money but only to help."[7]

The death of this young research subject, a participant in a gene therapy trial at the University of Pennsylvania, resulted in an investigation of possible conflicts of interest. The inquiry revealed perceived financial conflicts of a co-investigator.[8] The American Society of Gene Therapy then established a policy that prohibits all investigators and team members who are directly responsible for the selection of patients, the informed consent process, and/or clinical management in a trial from having equity, stock options, or comparable arrangements in companies that are sponsoring the trial.[9] Investigators must be seen as objective in their performance of clinical research. The data should be evaluated without taint of conflict of interest, or the integrity of the research will be at risk. There are all sorts of conflicts, and the degree to which each affects the objectivity of the researchers is relative. For example, some less obvious conflicts include possible career advancement through multiple publications and grant renewals.

In August 2000, NIH hosted a national conference, "Human Subjects Protection and Financial Conflicts of Interest," which lead to draft interim guidance.[10] Other recommendations and policy statements were issued by the Association of American Universities,[11] the National Bioethics Advisory Commission,[12] the American Medical Association,[13] and the International Committee of Medical Journal Editors (ICMJE).[14]

What Is a Reportable Conflict of Interest?

For the purposes of reporting to federal and institutional authorities, a *conflict of interest* is the existence of financial or personal interests that may influence the objectivity of the investigator and potentially influence the integrity of the research results.

Who Has to Report What, and to Which Agencies?

It would be simple if there was only one set of federal regulations to be used as guidance for all involved in the research process. Unfortunately, this is not the case. At least three agencies have issued conflict of interest guidelines and not all apply to all participants. Reporting obligations will be discussed here as they affect the investigative site (organization) and the sponsor; the reporting obligations of the IRBs will be discussed in chapter 8.

Investigative Site Reporting Obligations

The U.S. Public Health Service (PHS) has issued regulations that encompass projects funded by that agency only. All investigators and other involved individuals are subject to these regulations. This requirement extends to investigators' spouses and dependent children. The amount that must be reported is $10,000 or greater in ownership or interests in the company whose products are being tested, or any interest that may reasonably appear to affect the research. What interests would be considered as conflicts? Usually it is monetary, including, but not limited to, salary or other payments for services (for example, consulting fees or honoraria); equity interests (for example, stocks, stock options, or other ownership interests); and intellectual property rights (for example, patents, copyrights, and royalties from such rights).[15]

The reportable conflict of interests policy is applied to institutions as well. Institutions do not have to report the nature of the conflict of interest, but they must assure PHS that they will manage, reduce, or eliminate the conflict in accordance with the regulation. Institutions are given 60 days to report any conflicting interests that they identify after an initial report has been filed. The PHS recommends that teaching hospitals that accept research and education funding from the pharmaceuticals industry do not allow sponsors to offer gifts to investigators or students.[16]

How Are Institutions to "Manage" Conflict?

Under PHS regulations, institutions must establish guidelines and maintain a system to enforce these institutional policies. The institution must maintain a written policy that details how the conflict of interest (COI) policy is to be implemented and enforced. All financial disclosures must be reviewed and reported as above. If PHS regulations in this regard are not followed, funding will be discontinued.[17]

The National Science Foundation (NSF) has issued requirements that are similar to the PHS regulations. These apply to institutions that have more than 50 employees who receive NSF funding. The management of conflict is not as concise as the NSF requirements may seem to suggest, however. In addition, reporting to the Office of General Counsel of the NSF is only required if the conflict has not been "satisfactorily managed."[18]

21 *CFR* 54 states that investigators must report conflicts or changes in conflicts for a period of time (from study start-up to end of trial—defined as first database lock plus one year). The sponsor is not obligated to solicit this information, but may remind investigators of this requirement.

What if the Investigator or the Institution Is the Sponsor of the Research Performed with a New Pharmaceutical Agent or Device?

In the case of investigator-sponsored research, the FDA rules on conflict of interest apply, and the investigator or institution has the same reporting and compliance responsibilities as a sponsor does. These responsibilities are outlined immediately below in "The Sponsors' Reporting Responsibilities."

In the OHRP draft regarding conflict of interest (10 January 2001), the following are suggested for institutions. (1) A conflict of interests institutional official or committee should be selected to evaluate potential or real conflicts and their effect on the conduct and reporting of the proposed research. (2) Institutions must ensure that the IRB is free of institutional pressures. (3) If the institution is the sponsor, a separate and independent advisory and oversight committee should be established to assess the situation.

The Sponsors' Reporting Responsibilities

The FDA's Financial Disclosure regulation (21 *CFR* 54) applies to pharmaceutical companies, device manufacturers, and any other party that has applied for a marketing application for FDA approval. Institutions and investigators are not required to report any conflicts to the FDA directly, however, they must communicate their conflicts to the sponsor, who will then forward that information to the FDA. The forms to be submitted are FDA 3455, if there are any conflicts; or form 3454, in the case of no reportable conflicts.[19] (The PHS dollar threshold for reportable conflicts is higher—$25,000 of cumulative monetary value and $50,000 of equity interest in a publicly held company). The nature of the FDA requirement is somewhat different. The FDA is more interested in conflicts that may relate to the relationship between the investigator and the research sponsor, such as the relationship between study outcome and the value of the investigator's compensation, and whether the investigator has a proprietary interest in the product, such as a patent or licensing agreement. The sponsors must retain a file that records the financial interests of the investigators for at least two years after the date of application approval.

In 1994, the OIG issued a fraud alert in response to activity by pharmaceutical companies such as payments called "research grants" that were compensation for performing tasks for sponsors other than research. Typically this would include "studies" in which a physician uses an approved agent for an approved labeling of the drug and is paid some sum of money to report on the patient's satisfaction with the product. This type of activity is not considered legitimate scientific research.[20] IRBs and conflicts of interest are covered in chapter 8.

In summary, there are numerous regulations that address financial and conflict of interest issues in clinical research. At times it is difficult to ascertain what and when to report to which agency. For the future, it is reasonable to anticipate additional or changing requirements and increasing amounts of federal oversight of the financial aspects of human research.

5.4 TAKE AWAY MESSAGES

- Educational and quality assurance requirements have substantially increased the costs of running a human subjects protections program.
- Organizations must provide sufficient financial and organizational support for human subjects protections efforts.
- Determinants of needed staff include number of actions processed, the number of new protocols reviewed, and the frequency of meetings.
- Consider cost sharing among all involved—organizations, sponsors, and investigators.
- Many conflicts of interest are financial, but others are nonfinancial, and offer other possibilities for personal gain.
- Organizations must wrestle with sometimes confusing guidelines from various agencies to ensure that they are managing any real or perceived conflicts of interest.
- IRBs must be insulated from institutional pressures.

NOTES

1. Johns Hopkins University: S. Levine and R. Weiss, "Hopkins Told to Halt Trials Funded by U.S.; Death of Medical Volunteer Prompted Federal Directive," *Washington Post*, 20 July 2001; J. Bor and T. Pelton, "US Halts Hopkins Research: Most Experiments on Human Subjects Ordered Suspended, Federal Funding Withheld, Oversight Agency Decries Safety Lapses in Volunteer's Death," *Baltimore Sun*, 20 July 2001; "Funds Halted after Asthma Death," *Toronto Star*, 20 July 2001; A. Dembner, "Human Test at Hopkins Halted," *Boston Globe*, 20 July 2001.

Duke University: J.B. Obermayer and S. Cauffman, "US Halts Human Clinical Trials at Duke," *News and Observer*, 12 May 1999; T. Monmaney, "Safety Concerns Suspend Research at Duke Hospital," *Wilmington (N.C.) Morning Star*, 12 May 1999.

The Charles R. Drew University and Science Center and its affiliate, Martin Luther King Jr. Hospital in California: N. Riccardi and T. Monmaney, "King/Drew Medical Research Suspended Health: Voluntary Action Comes After Regulators Find Two Dozen Violations of Rules Designed to Protect Human Subjects and Insurance Credibility at South LA Facility," *Los Angeles Times*, 27 April 2000.

2. DHHS, *http://oig.hhs.gov/oei/reports/oei-01-97-00197.pdf*, accessed 10 July 2002.

3. See note 1 above.

4. Bioethics Resources on the web, NIH, *http://www.nih.gov/sigs/bioethics/IRB.html*, accessed 22 April 2002.

5. DHHS, "Report of the Office of In-

spector General; Institutional Review Boards—A Time for Reform," *http://oig.hhs.gov/oei/reports/a276.pdf*, accessed 10 July 2002.

6. See note 1 above.

7. *Gelsinger v. University of Pennsylvania*, Philadelphia County Court of Common Pleas, Term 2000 (complaint filed 19 September 2000; settled 4 November 2000).

8. Ibid.

9. American Society of Gene Therapy, *Policy Statement*, 5 April 2000, *http://www.asgt.org/policy/*, accessed 21 April 2002.

10. *Draft Interim Guidance*, 10 January 2001, *http://ohrp.osophs.dhhs.gov/nhrpac/mtg12-00/finguid.htm*, accessed 21 April 2002.

11. Association of American Universities, Task Force on Research Accountability, "Report on Individual and Institutional Financial Conflict of Interest," October 2001, *http://www.aau.edu/research/COI.01.pdf*, accessed 15 July 2002.

12. National Bioethics Advisory Commission, *Ethical and Policy Issues in Research Involving Human Participants* (Bethesda, Md.: National Bioethics Advisory Commission, August 2001).

13. The current statement by the American Medical Association on conflicts of interest is AMA Council on Scientific Affairs, Influence of Funding Source on Outcome, Validity, and Reliability of Pharmaceutical Research, June 2004, *http://www.ama-assn.org/ama/pub/article/2036-8608.html*, accessed 15 July 2004.

14. International Committee of Medical Journal Editors, "II. Ethical Considerations in the Conduct and Reporting of Research. D. Conflicts of Interest," *Uniform Requirements for Manuscripts Submitted to Biomedical Journals: Writing and Editing for Biomedical Publication*, *http://www.icmje.org/index.html*, accessed 15 July 2004.

15.42 *CFR* 50, Subpart F.

16. 42 *CFR* 50.604.

17. 5 *CFR* Part 2635; 5 *CFR* Part 2635; 5 *CFR* Part 5301; 5 *CFR* Part 2634.

18. See note 10 above.

19. 21 *CFR* 54.4a.

20. DHHS, *//oig.hhs.gov/fraud/docs/alertsandbulletins/121994.html, accessed 10 July 2002.*

6

Education and Human Subject Protections

Deirdre Hall, CCRC, CCRA, CIP

Protecting human research subjects is a complex mission. Education is essential and has always been the right thing to do. Now it is also mandated. This chapter will cover these topics.

6.1 BACKGROUND AND BASICS

Protecting human subjects is not solely the responsibility of the IRB. It is the responsibility of every person and organization that conducts research with human subjects. As this is the case, each of these parties must understand their responsibilities. Education that is focused on human subjects protections must include investigators, research staff, nursing staff, IRB members, and sponsor staff. Education is one of the greatest means of effecting change. It is also critically important in an environment where regulations and guidelines change, and research consciousness is raised through experience. While "basic" training in the conduct of human experimentation is imperative, continuing education is also essential. The goal of most educational programs should be to enhance the abilities of the responsible parties to carry out their roles by developing their skills, and increasing their knowledge and motivation.

The times have changed rapidly, as is evidenced by a quote from Dr. Louis Lasagna of the Center for the Study of Drug Development at Tufts University. In 1991, Dr. Lasagna wrote, in a foreword to Bert Spilker's text, *Guide to Clinical Trials*,

> Equally clear is the fact that the formal training of basic scientists, physicians,

dentists, veterinarians, pharmacists, nurses, statisticians, etc. does little to prepare these individuals for careers in pharmaceutical development and regulation. It is not necessary to deny categorically the utility of such formal training to conclude that the training is inevitably woefully inadequate for such careers. For the near future at least, 'on the job training' will be the order of the day, with self-teaching an important component.[1]

The Bottom Line

Educational programs should cover numerous topics in the responsible conduct of human research and should offer a variety of educational formats to cater to different individuals. Programs should provide students with general training as well as area-specific training. Institutions and other research organizations should establish educational and training policies.

Is This Just a Nice Idea?

Organizations are being held accountable for ensuring that research professionals are qualified to perform research activities. The Office of Human Research Protection (OHRP) expects human subjects protection administrators, IRB staff, and institutional officials to be educated in human subjects protection and the ethics of human subject research.[2] During an IRB inspection, OHRP looks for educational programs that demonstrate that IRB members have been trained, but also that investigators have been appropriately informed.[3] FDA surely looks to ensure that the staff of a chosen investigational site has been trained and is appropriately qualified on multiple levels.[4]

The Association for the Accreditation of Human Research Protection Programs (AAHRPP) Accreditations Standards support the need for education: the first two principles of Accreditation of Human Research Protection Programs, as defined by AAHRPP, are, in fact,

> 1. Regulatory compliance is a minimal expectation for a human research protection program. 2. Protecting the rights and welfare of human research participants must be a research organization's first priority. Beyond assessing compliance with applicable regulations, accreditation standards should promote a research environment where ethical, productive investigation is valued.[5]

Most institutions and organizations now recognize that education is a direct and meaningful way to ensure the protection of human research subjects.

6.2 ARE THERE EDUCATION REQUIREMENTS?

Yes. In 2001, the National Institutes of Health (NIH) established an education requirement for human subject research.[6] The requirement applies to all projects that receive NIH support after 1 October 2000. All individuals must document that they have completed an educational program on the protection of human research participants. This requirement applies to all individuals who are involved in the design, conduct, or reporting of research.

More important than the *requirements* for training and education is a change in philosophy: that education about human subjects protection helps to ensure subjects' safety. Training and education should extend beyond IRB members and include other clinical research professionals—both from academia and industry—and the subjects of research, too.

The AAHRPP accreditation standards indicate the expectations that institutions will protect human subjects. These standards do not only apply to NIH-funded research. This is important, as many institutions that conduct human subject research will never conduct NIH-funded research. There is a recurrent problem of too little guidance about the most effective means of achieving the minimum standards of regulations. Thus, OHRP accreditation standards are worth repeating here:

> The organization ensures that all personnel reviewing, conducting or supporting human research (including IRB members and personnel involved in the Human Research Protection Program) demonstrate sufficient knowledge of the protection of research participants.
>
> The organization uses policies, procedures, and *education programs* to help its investigators carry out research studies ethically. In addition to following applicable federal, state, and local regulations, investigators follow ethical principles and standards appropriate for their discipline. In designing and conducting clinical trials, investigators follow Good Clinical Practice guidelines defined by the Food and Drug Administration. In designing and conducting all research studies, investigators have as the primary concern protecting the rights and welfare of participants [emphasis added].[7]

6.3 CREATING YOUR OWN TRAINING PROGRAM

Training people in good clinical research practice can be a daunting task. What will it take to do it effectively? Several things: (1) talented instructors who are enthusiastic and knowledgeable about clinical research, good clinical practice (GCP), and human research subject protection; (2) clearly defined objectives, and (3) interactive instruction with multiple media. Some good motivational tools are food (that is: lunch, pizza, donuts); the chance to earn contact hours/continuing medical education credits also goes a long way to motivating students. Management "buy-in" is also critical; educational initiatives need to be supported from the top down. Let's address each of these items.

What Makes an Instructor Excellent?

Reviewing regulations, standard operating procedures (SOPs), and rules is not ordinarily a "fun" way to pass time. An excellent instructor will make such review stimulating through good verbal skills, interpersonal skills, and an extensive knowledge of the subject matter. Later in this chapter, we will explore techniques that can help the non-teacher—yet enthusiastic clinical research professional—be a great trainer.

What are Clearly Defined Objectives, and Why are They Important?

Tell students what they can expect to learn from a training session. The assessment of objectives that have been met is a good barometer for whether the instructor did the job. A list of objectives assists trainees in choosing the appropriate training courses. Such lists help to keep students interested as they cross-check to determine whether various learning objectives have been met. Objectives also keep the instructor focused on the appropriate material.

Why Does the Training Have to Be Interactive?

Many students dislike participating in public training sessions, but it's important to work past that concern in the interest of having a more productive learning opportunity. Engaging people in conversation, debate, and mock activities are ways to keep interest in the subject matter and will help to ensure and gauge whether the message is getting across. This is active rather than passive learning.

Multiple Speakers Keep Interest

Frequently, training agendas are lengthy. It is difficult for students and instructors to keep interest if only one instructor is assigned to the program. Rotate lecturers or break up sessions with other media such as videos. The OHRP distributes a video, "Protection of Human Subjects," which includes an overview of *The Belmont Report* that can be a useful addition to an orientation program.[8] A CD-ROM is also available through OHRP and PRIM&R (Public Responsibility in Medicine & Research) entitled "Investigator-101."[9]

What Other Techniques Are Useful?

The instructor should carefully consider the handouts that are provided to students. Keep it simple. It is often helpful to distribute copies of a PowerPoint presentation and other reference materials. Many instructors prefer to distribute bulleted lists of the key items of their presentation.

6.4 CHOOSING COURSE CONTENT

Choosing course content comes naturally to some teachers. Developing workshops becomes easier with experience. A great instructor thinks through several steps when designing a program. The first step is to identify the audience. Once the characteristics of the audience have been determined, the rest of the process falls into place. An educator must consider the allotted time frame, whether the program is mandatory or voluntary, and the size and knowledge level of the audience. A needs assessment should be performed to guide the instructor. Program organizers should consider the following types of questions: What are the needs of the workshop participants? Have previous audits demonstrated that informed consent documents are routinely deficient? Is the IRB consistently having difficulty approving projects due to insufficient information from the investigator? These are all items that provide information on the needs of the audience and research community at large.

There are numerous other ways to choose topics for educational activities and to stay abreast of current trends in clinical research. Some excellent choices include participating in several listservs, including OHRP, NIH, FDA, and the IRB Forum (see "Useful Websites" at the end of this book). There are numerous periodicals that are useful as well. These include FDA warning letters and OHRP determination letters available to the public under the Freedom of Information Act (FOIA). Others include *Human Research Report*, *IRB Advisor*, *IRB—Ethics and Human Research*, *Medical Ethics Advisor*, and *Research Practitioner*. Memberships in organizations are also useful. Important organizations include the following:

- Association for Clinical Research Professionals (ACRP),
- Applied Research Ethics National Association (ARENA),
- Drug Information Association (DIA),
- Pharmaceutical Manufacturers of America (PhRMA),
- Public Responsibility in Research and Medicine (PRIM&R),
- Society of Clinical Research Associates (SoCRA), and
- Society of Quality Assurance (SQA).

Please refer to the list of valuable websites included at the end of this book.

Some industry sponsors have created positions for IRB liaisons to help foster the educational and interactive processes between industry sponsors and IRB professionals.[10]

Other General Tips

Teaching any subject requires instructors to be innovative, creative, and persistent. Teachers should provide opportunities to problem solve and apply the principles being taught. Case studies are very effective in achieving this goal. Sometimes one-on-one training is what is needed: monitors teach coordinators at the investigational site; IRB administrators teach investigators good clinical practice when an unusual situation arises and the investigator calls to inquire; IRBs and sponsors learn from each other during dispute resolution regarding an informed consent document. It happens all the time. And while such learning experiences do not replace the need for formalized training, they are invaluable.

It is important to recognize that we must be educators. The old method of clinical research training, which usually consisted of baptism by fire, is no longer acceptable. Education about the protection of human subjects must be rigorous and continuous. All clinical research professionals have an obligation to mentor, stay informed, and share knowledge and resources.

What Does "Continuing Education" Mean?

This aspect of training and education can often be the most difficult. An annual workshop that reviews basic human subjects protection issues is probably not enough. Many IRBs provide some continuing education at each IRB meeting. The administrator or chair who organizes these efforts needs to identify timely topics, perhaps compile reading materials or other references, and prepare a short overview, usually presented at the time of the convened meeting. It is easy for the continuing education component to get glossed over if there is a large agenda. Herein lies the difficulty of providing continuing education in this setting.

There is no firm *requirement* for continuing education of IRB members, but there is a firm expectation of continuing education. The OHRP

> strongly recommends that the Institution and the designated IRB(s) establish educational training and oversight mechanisms (appropriate to the nature and volume of its research) to ensure that research investigators, IRB members and staff, and other appropriate personnel maintain continuing knowledge of, and comply with, relevant ethical principles, relevant Federal Regulations, OHRP guidance, other applicable guidance, state and local laws, and institutional policies for the protection of human subjects. Furthermore, OHRP recommends that a) IRB members and staff complete relevant educational training before reviewing human subject research; and b) research investigators complete appropriate institutional educational training before conducting human subject research.[11]

Some IRB administrators will prepare summaries of recent related literature or will write newsletters with updated information. These approaches are often successful, but don't incorporate the interactive component so critical to the IRB process in general.

Sponsors and other organizations have similar difficulties. How does one bring together large groups of clinical research professionals on a routine basis to impart new (or sometimes repetitive) information? These are busy professionals we are talking about! The most successful solution to this dilemma is to include continuing education as an organization's core value. Support for continuing education should come from the top down in any organization. It can be required and should be documented. Records of continuing education should be reviewed at the time of an employee's performance assessment.

What Should Be the Core Content for a Basic Human Subjects Protections Education Program?

Organizations should embrace a long-term commitment to providing high quality and relevant instruction to clinical research professionals. Once this has been effected, the core content of the program should be instated to ensure a baseline of knowledge at the organization.

Core content areas often include historical perspectives of human subjects protection, ethical issues in human subjects research—*The Nuremberg Code,*[12] *The Declaration of Helsinki,*[13] *The Belmont Report;*[14] investigator, IRB and sponsor obligations; an overview of IRB authority; issues in the conduct of research in vulnerable populations; and the principles of good clinical practice and informed consent. The Office for Research Integrity's[15] overview on the Responsible Conduct of Research suggests additional content, including data acquisition; management, sharing, and ownership of data; research misconduct; and conflicts of interest.

Additionally, clinical research professionals should be comfortable referencing the *Code of Federal Regulations* (*CFR*),the International Conference on Harmonisation (ICH)[16] *Good Clinical Practice Guidelines,* and other guidance documents. Teaching researchers about various resources and their content is an essential component of all training programs. All other training programs can progress from these core content areas.

6.5 TOOLS FOR EDUCATIONAL PROGRAMS

The November 2001 issue of *IRB Advisor* headlined: "Good News: there's more than one way to meet new educational requirements."[17] A variety of tools are now available to facilitate the learning process. Web-based learning is an increasingly popular way to reach groups who may be unable to travel to a course. Users of web-based learning can access an educational module at a time that is convenient to them and review materials at their own pace. However, there are drawbacks to web-based learning initiatives. First, some users have a difficult time learning via reading and review on a computer. Further, not all users will have access to the equipment necessary for viewing the educational program.

Other tools include CD-ROMs that can be easily and inexpensively distributed to those who need training. Videoconferencing courses allow interaction from a remote location. As previously mentioned, videos are an option for communicating information. Role-playing, games, simulations, and case studies are popular approaches incorporated into workshops.

Measuring understanding is an integral part of any training program. Measurement surveys/self assessment instruments, pre-tests and post-tests are all techniques for measuring comprehension. Repetition of information in these contexts can also be a useful means of learning.

The Beecher exposés, published in the *New England Journal of Medicine* in 1966,[18] are an excellent tool for facilitating discussion with all levels of clinical research professionals. They serve as an excellent backdrop for understanding the rationale and increased scrutiny of the research community. The exposés support the need for regulation and oversight in these activities. Modern case studies are excellent training tools as well.

6.6 STAYING ABREAST

Learn from Others' Mistakes—Know the Common Pitfalls

Under the Freedom of Information Act (FOIA), both OHRP and FDA make records of compliance activities available to the public. The OHRP has a section on its website entitled "Determination Letters." The FDA has a Freedom of Information Electronic Reading Room, where warning letters across all FDA divisions and oversight areas are posted. Information under FOIA is also available to the general public, if it is requested in writing. These web addresses can be found in Appendix B.

Clinical research professionals should learn from the experiences of others. The Determination Letters and FDA warning letters are important correspondence that provide insight into current trends, common compliance issues, and deficiencies. Why not use another organization's learning experience to improve or enhance our own processes, systems, or policies in the protection of human subjects?

View Other Educational Programs

Numerous organizations have written and designed superb educational programs. Access to many of these is available online. Most organizations share their programs or sell them to other organizations. Several universities now offer certificate, undergraduate, and graduate programs in clinical research or biomedical research ethics.

Hire a Consultant or Professional Trainer

There are also organizations that provide trainers or offer training workshops. It is sometimes more interesting and economical to invite speakers from other organizations.

What are Other Organizations Doing?

Some organizations have established educational branches or divisions that emphasize training in human subjects protection teaching. Many offer continuing education. For research compliance purposes, some institutions require investigators and other research professionals to earn a certain number of credits each year. Still other organizations require that students complete and pass exams at the end of each training program.

An important step is to write a continuing education policy that directs all continuing education at the local level. The policy should describe acceptable continuing education activities. For example, attendance at IRB meetings, local courses, or web-based training programs that deal with human subjects protection meet the policy requirements of some organizations. Policy can dictate how frequently investigators and other clinical research professionals show evidence of taking continuing education training.

Some IRBs are farther ahead in their training and general understanding of human subjects protection principles than others, which accounts for some of the differences in how IRBs approach the various projects they review.

Summing Up

The National Bioethics Advisory Commission sums the issue up in its report, "Ethical and Policy Issues in Research Involving Human Participants," published in August 2001.

> It is unrealistic to think that ethical obligations can be fully met without guidance and resources. *To help researchers and IRBs fulfill their responsibilities, the federal government should promote the development of education, certification, and accreditation systems that apply to all researchers, all IRB members and staff, and all institutions [emphasis added].* These tools should help researchers craft, and IRBs review, studies that pose few problems, and to know

when their work requires special oversight. Today, investigators and IRBs are rightly confused about issues as basic as which areas of inquiry should be reviewed and who constitutes a human participant.

Education is the foundation of the oversight system and is essential to protecting research participants. In all of our reports, we have highlighted the need to educate all those involved in research with human participants, including the public, investigators, IRB members, institutions, and federal agencies.[19]

6.7 SAMPLE TOPICS FOR EDUCATIONAL PROGRAMS IN CLINICAL ETHICS

- Identifying and Managing Conflicts of Interest in Clinical Research
- Practical Challenges of Informed Consent in Clinical Trials
- Research or Practice?
- Role of the IRB in Assuring Responsible Conduct of Research
- New Directions in Research Ethics
- HIPAA and its Implications for Human Subject Research
- Legally Acceptable Representatives and Research
- Placebo Controls in Clinical Trials
- Managing Sponsor/Investigator Relations
- Expectation Management—Partnering with other Clinical Research Professionals
- Applying the Principles of *The Belmont Report*
- Statistics for the Non-Statistician
- Surviving a Federal Inspection
- Updates on the Federal Regulations
- "Lunch and Learn" to Review Warning and Determination Letters
- Therapeutic Overviews and Implications in Human Subject Research
- Gene Transfer Research: Interaction between the IRB and institutional biosafety committees (IBCs)
- How to Write Standard Operating Procedures
- Project Management Tips
- Understanding the Organization's Standard Operating Procedures
- Implications of Electronic Submissions Regulations (21 *CFR* 11)
- The Trial is Approved . . . What's Next?
- The IRB Liaison—Interactions between Sponsors and IRBs

6.8 SAMPLE EDUCATIONAL OBJECTIVES FOR PROGRAMS

At the conclusion of this activity, participants should be able to:

- Discuss fundamental concepts and principles for understanding the ethics of research with humans.
- Describe the mechanism of review of research proposals involving humans and current federal regulations pertaining to research with humans.
- Chronicle the history of ethical issues associated with research with humans
- Identify emerging issues in research with humans and develop possible approaches for considering and addressing those issues.
- Follow the literature on ethical issues associated with human subjects research.
- Implement skills in evaluating research proposals involving humans.
- Describe the basic ethical and regulatory expectations regarding integrity in clinical research.
- Identify strategies for improving individual and institutional practices regarding data acquisition and handling.
- Recognize and remediate deficiencies associated with subject recruitment and informed consent, conflict of interest, and compliance with research integrity

and human subjects protection standards.
- Identify investigator obligations under 21 *CFR* 312 and 812 and ICH.
- Evaluate adverse events and adhere to reporting requirements and timelines
- Understand the role of the IRB, research coordinator, sponsor, contract research organizations (CROs), and clinical research associates (CRAs).
- Define common clinical research terms
- Effectively conduct a consent interview
- Discuss historical perspectives of clinical research and research reform.
- Protect personal data privacy while conducting a clinical trial.

6.9 SAMPLE PROGRAM SYLLABI[20]

Why Do Clinical Research?
- Positives and Negatives of Conducting Clinical Trials
- Historical Perspectives of Clinical Research and Research Reform
- Common Themes in the History of Human Subjects Research
- Chronology of the Evolution of Clinical Research Regulations
- *The Nuremberg Code, The Declaration of Helsinki* and *The Belmont Report*
- Henry Beecher's Exposés
- Tuskegee Experiment, Willowbrook, Jewish Chronic Disease Hospital, San Antonio Contraceptive Trial, Tea Room Trade, and Obedience to Authority
- Common Deficiencies at the Investigational Site
  - As noted by FDA
  - As noted by OHRP Biomedical Research Fraud Federal Oversight Inspections
- What Inspectors Look For
- Investigators' Responsibilities
  - As defined in 21 *CFR* 312 and 812 and in the International Conference on Harmonisation's Good Clinical Practice Guidelines
  - Issues regarding Delegation of Authority Federal Regulations, GCP, and ICH
  - Applicability and general content
  - 21 *CFR* 11, 50, 54, 56, 312, 314, 812, 814, 600
  - 5 *CFR* 46
  - ICH *GCP Guideline* May 1996

Institutional Review Boards
- Purpose
- Membership Requirements
- Procedures, Reporting Requirements, and Authority
- Partnering with the IRB

Informed Consent
- Document and Process
- Procedures for Obtaining Informed Consent
- Required Elements of Informed Consent
- Differences between DHHS, FDA, and ICH Regarding Informed Consent
- Documenting Informed Consent
- Exceptions from the Informed Consent Requirement
- Assent
- Legally Acceptable Representative

Conduct of Studies
- Recognizing and Reporting Adverse Events
- Essential documents
- Subject "Case Histories" and record keeping
- Record Retention Requirements
- Case Report Forms Versus Source Documents
- Ethically Recruiting Research Subjects
- Clinical Trial "Walk-Through"
  - Outline of the Various Steps and Sponsor Driven Activities that Occur During a Clinical Trial
- Subject Follow Up and Compliance

Sample Program Syllabus
Basic IRB Training for IRB Members and Staff, Investigators, Research Sponsors,

and Other Clinical Research Professionals[21]

- Today's Scrutiny of IRBs: What Is the Buzz About?
  - Discussion of suspensions, lessons learned, results of suspensions, summary of major noncompliance issues
- So History Shall Not Repeat Itself: Historical Perspectives of Clinical Research and Research Reform
  - Overview of the historical precedent for IRBs, research "tragedies" (for example, thalidomide, sulfanilamide, Tuskegee Experiment, Willowbrook, Medical War Crimes of World War II), historical research ethics documents, and current implications for IRBs (*The Nuremberg Code*, *The Declaration of Helsinki*, and *The Belmont Report*)
- Who Has the Answers?
  - Overview of Federal Regulations and Policies for Human Subject Protections, IRB Authority and Composition, Mechanisms of Review/Types of Review, Criteria for IRB Approval, Reporting/Record Keeping Requirements
- Informed Consent: Document and Process: What's Gone Wrong?
  - Common Findings of Noncompliance
  - Review of the Common OHRP Findings; an IRBs Responsibility to Audit Investigators
  - Why an IRB Should Inspect Investigational Sites
  - What Should IRB Auditors Look For?
- Human Subjects Smorgasbord
  - IRB Record Keeping: What Should You Have in Your IRB Policies and Procedures
  - Continuing Review Obligations
  - Meeting Minutes
  - Fulfilling Continuing Education Obligations for Investigators and IRB Members/Chairs/Staff
  - IRBs and the Genetics Revolution
- What's on the Horizon?
  - Questions and Answers

6.10 SAMPLE EVALUATION/ FEEDBACK TOOL

Figure 6.10 presents a sample evaluation/feedback tool.[22]

6.11 TAKE AWAY MESSAGES

- Sponsors and institutions are obligated to ensure that their staff are educated in human subjects protection issues.
- There are numerous tools and creative approaches for fulfilling continuing education needs.
- Protecting human subjects is not solely the responsibility of the IRB. All clinical research professionals have an obligation to get informed and stay informed about good clinical practices.
- We are all teachers of good clinical practices—some in a direct way, others in an indirect way.
- Core content areas often include historical perspectives of human subjects protection, ethical issues in human subjects research (*The Nuremberg Code*, *The Declaration of Helsinki*, *The Belmont Report*), investigator, IRB and sponsor obligations, an overview of IRB authority, issues in conducting research in vulnerable populations, and the principles of good clinical practice and informed consent.
- In 2000, the NIH established an education requirement for human subject research. The requirement applies to all projects that receive NIH support after 1 October 2000.

NOTES

1. L. Lasagna, "Foreword," in *Guide to Clinical Trials,* B. Spilker (Philadelphia, Pa.: Lippincott, Williams & Wilkins, 1991).

Evaluation/Feedback Tool

Date: ______________________ **Course Title:** ______________________
Name of Instructor: ______________________

Scale:
1 = Excellent, 2 = Very good, 3 = Good, 4 = Fair, 5 = Poor, 6 = Not applicable

Evaluation Criteria Score (see scale above)

- Mastery of subject ___
- Preparation for class ___
- Organization of material ___
- Presentation of material ___
- Ability to motivate students ___
- Ability to answer questions and channel discussion ___
- Use of blackboard/visual aids ___
- Attitude of instructor toward students ___
- Availability for consultation ___
- Approaches teaching with enthusiasm ___
- Provides students with opportunities to practice problem-solving skills ___
- Overall ability as a teacher ___

Location of Physical Facilities:

- Facilities (overall) ___
- Classroom temperature ___
- Restrooms ___
- Refreshments ___
- Lighting ___
- Audiovisual equipment ___
- Accessibility ___

Quality of Program Materials:

- Manuals ___
- Handouts ___

Did this Program (circle Yes or No):

- Adequately outline communications with Institutional Review Boards? Yes No
- Offer guidance in the ethical recruitment of research subjects? Yes No
- Teach you how to prepare for sponsor visits? Yes No
- Give you a better understanding of the various phases of clinical trials? Yes No
- Give you a better understanding of research terminology? Yes No
- Teach you about the *Code of Federal Regulations* (that is, which regulations govern particular aspects of clinical research activities)? Yes No
- Provide clearly defined objectives? Yes No
- Help you to better be able to manage your responsibilities as a research coordinator? Yes No
- Help you feel more prepared to conduct an informed consent conversation since taking this course? Yes No
- Help you in identifying adverse events more readily? Yes No
- Give you a perspective of the history of clinical research? Yes No
- Help you better understand the roles of each member of the clinical research team? Yes No
- Help you to manage necessary documentation specific to clinical trials? Yes No

Comments:

____

____

Figure 6.10. Sample evaluation/feedback tool for educational programs.

2. OHRP, 4 April 2002, Item 50, *http://ohrp.osophs.dhhs.gov/references/finding.pdf,* accessed 2 July 2002.

3. Ibid.

4. FDA Information Sheets, "Self-Evaluation Checklist for IRBs," *http://www.fda.gov/oc/ohrt/irbs/irbchecklist.html,* accessed 2 July 2002.

5. Association for the Accreditation of Human Research Protection Programs, "Principles and Standards," *http://www.aahrpp.org/principles.htm,* accessed 26 June 2002.

6. "Required Education in the Protection Of Human Research Participants," release date 5 September 2001, National Institutes of Health, *http://grants2.nih.gov/grants/guide/notice-files/NOT-OD-01-061.html,* accessed 26 June 2002.

7. See note 5 above.

8. Videotape series, *Protection of Human Subjects*, available through the Office for Human Research Protections, *http://ohrp.orophs.dhhs.gov/references/resource.htm,* accessed 1 July 2002.

9. "Investigator 101—Office for Human Research Protections and Public Responsibility in Medicine and Research," *http://ohrp.osophs.dhhs.gov/references/cdrom.pdf,* accessed 1 July 2002.

10. Personal communication with Linda Simrell, MD, Merck Pharmaceuticals.

11. "Terms of the Federal Wide Assurance for Institutions within the United States," *http://ohrp.osophs.dhhs.gov/humansubjects/assurance/filasurt.htm,* accessed 2 July 2002.

12. *The Nuremberg Code,* "Permissible Medical Experiments," *Trials of War Criminals before the Nuernberg Military Tribunals under Control Council Law No. 10: Nuernberg, October 1946 -April 1949* (Washington, D.C.: U.S. Government Printing Office, n.d., vol. 2): 181-2; *http://ohsrod.nih.gov/nuremberg.php3,* accessed 10 July 2002.

13. World Medical Association, *The Declaration of Helsinki, http://www.wma.net/e/ethicsunit/helsinki.htm,* accessed 10 July 2004.

14. U.S. Department of Health, Education and Welfare, *The Belmont Report* (Washington, D.C.: U.S. Government Printing Office, 1988, 201/778-80319 GPO 887-809); originally published in 44 *Federal Register* (18 April 1979), 23192-7; *http://ohrp. osophs.dhhs.gov/human subjects/guidance/belmont.htm,* accessed 10 July 2002.

15. Office of Research Integrity, "Responsible Conduct of Research Education," *www.ori.dhhs.gov/html/programs/rce_requirements.asp,* accessed 10 July 2004.

16. ICH GCP Guidelines E6, *http://www.ifpma.org/pdf>ifpma/e6.pdf,* accessed 28 May 2002.

17. "Your Practical Guide to Institutional Review Board Management," *IRB Advisor* (November 2001), *www.ahcpub.com/ahc_root_html/products/newsletters/irb.html,* accessed 10 July 2004.

18. H.K. Beecher, "Ethics and Clinical Research," *New England Journal of Medicine,* 274 (1966):1354-60.

19. National Bioethics Advisory Commission, "Ethical and Policy Issues in Research Involving Human Participants," *http://bioethics.georgetown.edu/nbac/human/oversumm.pdf,* accessed 26 June 2002.

20. *Investigator Training Syllabus* (Great Neck, N.Y.: Biomedical Research Alliance of New York, Institute for Research Education, 2002).

21. D. Gutleber Hall, *Basic IRB Training Syllabus* (Great Neck, N.Y.: Biomedical Research Alliance of New York, Institute for Research Education, 2000).

22. D. Gutleber Hall, *Evaluate/Feedback Tool* (Great Neck, N.Y.: Biomedical Research Alliance of New York, Institute for Research Education, 1999).

7

The Role of Quality Assurance Reviews in Assuring Quality in Clinical Investigations

Kay Ryan, CIP, and Eileen Hilton, MD

Part A: Quality Assurance

Kay Ryan, CIP

This part of chapter 7 will highlight the following topics.

7.A.1 What Led to the Increase in Quality Assurance Efforts?
7.A.2 What an Investigator Should Expect from the QA Process
7.A.3 The QA Review Process
7.A.4 Interaction between the QA Specialist, the Investigator, and the Study Team
7.A.5 Take Away Messages

In the past five years we have seen heightened scrutiny of the clinical research enterprise by federal agencies, including the Office of the Inspector General (OIG), the General Accounting Office (GAO), the Office of Human Research Protection (OHRP), and the Food and Drug Administration (FDA); a number of national and international commissions; consumer advocate groups; and commercial sponsors.

The most recent trend is the promotion of self-assessments and quality assurance (QA) reviews. Contract research organizations (CROs) and sponsors regularly conduct QA audits of investigational sites, and some sponsors audit IRBs and other investigational sites. The FDA has a long standing Bioresearch Monitoring Program that monitors the performance of sponsors, monitors, and investigators, and the FDA performs QA on how it carries out its duties. In 2001, the FDA established an office for Good Clinical Practice (GCP) to coordinate activities within the agency to enhance protection of participants in research. In 2002, the OHRP announced a quality improvement program to help institutions evaluate and improve the quality of human research protections programs.[1] This initiative will assist IRBs in performing self-assessments and developing quality initiatives to achieve accreditation by private sector accrediting entities. Investigators and research organizations can glean valuable information from publicly available resources, including FDA warning letters and OHRP determination letters written to other parties.[2] Each of the major stakeholders in the clinical research enterprise—IRBs, sponsors, investigators, and research subjects—is affected by these process improvement initiatives.

7.A.1 WHAT LED TO THE INCREASE IN QUALITY ASSURANCE EFFORTS?

The reports generated by national commissions and the U.S. Department of Health and Human Services (DHHS) Office of the Inspector General have pointed out the large volume of studies that must be reviewed by the typical IRB, and the rather cursory reviews IRBs often give of applications to continue studies beyond the initial approval period.[3] Most IRBs have relied totally on information provided by investigators in approving continuation of protocols beyond their initial approval period. Few IRBs have conducted audits to ascertain investigators' adherence to approved protocols, appropriate reporting of unanticipated adverse events, and so forth. IRBs have been cited for allowing studies to continue in the absence of substantive and meaningful review.[4] Some IRBs have initiated QA review and continuous quality assurance and improvement programs based on this criticism, as well as on the statutory authority contained in documents published by the U.S. Department of Health and Human Services (DHHS), the FDA, and the International Conference on Harmonisation (ICH).[5]

The overarching objective of these audit/QA initiatives is to assure the safety of subjects through an assessment of how well investigators comply with the principles of GCPs.[6] The more focused objective of QA audits is to assure the integrity of the data that is generated in clinical trials which depends on adherence to protocols.

IRB Quality Assurance Initiatives

Many IRB-directed QA reviews are conducted as part of an IRB's education programs that are directed to investigators and study staff. Investigators benefit from a QA review in many ways, not the least of which is learning the extent to which a study is being performed in compliance with GCPs, identifying correctable deficiencies early in the study, and highlighting areas where additional staff training is appropriate.

Selection of Trials to be Audited

IRBs may select studies for QA review based on a number of factors, including the involvement of potentially vulnerable populations in the protocol, the number of subjects enrolled in the study, how long a study has been ongoing, the number of protocol amendments, the number of serious unexpected adverse events, consent form revisions, et cetera. The IRB may ask its QA specialist to observe the consent process. In addition, a study may be selected for review if it was terminated by the IRB because the approval period expired without any communication from the investigator that requested continuing approval or that notified the IRB of the closure of the study. A study may be selected for review "for cause"—as the result of a complaint from a subject or colleague, or as result of litigation (for example, subpoenas, discovery, and the like).

Investigators whose studies have received significant negative findings in previous audits (such as protocol violations and/or deviations, use of a consent form other than one that was approved by the IRB, failure to report serious and unexpected adverse events, et cetera) should expect more frequent QA reviews. In such instances, the investigator should approach the QA review process and the IRB's recommendations as a benchmark for meeting GCP standards and as a learning opportunity.

7.A.2 WHAT AN INVESTIGATOR SHOULD EXPECT FROM THE QA PROCESS

An IRB's QA review can provide an independent confirmation that a study was conducted in accordance with GCP.

A wide variety of professionals perform QA audits—physicians, pharmacists, nurses, clinical research associates—but the common denominator is their knowledge of the regulatory requirements for conducting investigations and experience in dealing with unforeseen issues that can arise during the conduct of studies. QA professionals perform their duties in accordance with written procedures that should be designed to provide the investigator with the maximum benefit from the QA process. Investigators should have a thorough understanding of how QA reviews will proceed.

The IRB QA program should have written standard operating procedures (SOPs) that should be shared with the investigator(s) prior to the beginning of the review. The SOPs should be sufficiently detailed to cover the general aspects of clinical investigations and should be supplemented by procedures that are applicable to the study being reviewed. It is important that the auditor's SOP cover the policy on distributing the final QA reports within the institution or to board members, as well as the institutional policy on maintaining the confidentiality of information contained in the QA final reports.

How Are Deficiencies Handled?

The investigator should have a clear understanding of the IRB's procedures for dealing with findings of serious deficiencies in the conduct of the study and/or harm to study subjects. The Department of Health and Human Services (DHHS) regulations require IRBs to have written procedures for ensuring prompt reporting to the IRB, to institutional officials, and to federal agencies of unanticipated problems involving risks to subjects or others, or any serious or continuing noncompliance with federal regulations. In addition, FDA and International Conference on Harmonisation (ICH) regulations (4.1.2) require the investigator/institution to inform study subjects about termination of the study, to assure that subjects receive appropriate therapy and follow up, and to provide a detailed written explanation for the suspension or termination to regulatory authorities and to the study sponsor. The information provided to the investigator should detail the IRB's procedure for suspending or terminating IRB approval of the investigation when a study is not being conducted in accordance with the IRB's requirements or when the study has been associated with unexpected, serious harm to subjects. IRBs are required to provide a written statement of their reasons for this action. The suspension or termination must be reported to the investigator, institutional officials, and federal agency officials.

7.A.3 THE QA REVIEW PROCESS

The IRB QA specialist should contact the investigator at least a week in advance of a proposed review date to schedule a mutually convenient time for the audit. In addition, the QA specialist should provide, in writing, detailed information on the scope of the audit, and a list of documents that the investigator should have on hand for review. A QA specialist may ask to monitor the consent process and/or review patients' charts, and "essential documents" (protocol-related documents that form the core of information about how the study was conducted, as well as the personnel who performed various aspects of the investigation) for compliance with federal and institutional policies. The QA specialist should provide the investigator with the IRB's QA program SOP, and the SOP should address the extent to which the IRB maintains the confidentiality of the final QA report.

The QA specialist should review the IRB's file (approved protocol, correspondence with the investigator, approved consent forms, protocol amendments, reports of adverse events, and so forth) prior to meeting with the investigator and the study team. The QA review generally focuses on a review of the essential documents; subject source documents should be reviewed for data verification.

Essential documents may include the following (when applicable):

1. Curricula vitae for the principal investigator and all listed sub-investigators (including non-physicians).
2. Completed, signed, and dated Form FDA 1571 (if the study is being conducted under a physician-investigational new drug—IND—protocol).
3. Completed, signed, and dated Form FDA 1572 (if the study is being conducted under an IND).
4. Signed protocol approval (signed by the investigator).
5. Signed protocol amendment approvals, if applicable.
6. IRB approval letter.
7. IRB approval letters for protocol amendments, if applicable.
8. IRB-approved informed consent form (current and previous versions, if any).
9. IRB membership roster.
10. License for local laboratory (if a local laboratory is used and a license is required by law) or certification for that laboratory.
11. Laboratory reference ranges (for local laboratories).
12. Drug shipment documentation: receipts, orders, returns, handling of drugs to subsites, et cetera.
13. Correspondence: IRB-investigator, sponsor-investigator, investigator-subject/patient.
14. Sponsor's monitoring reports.
15. Telephone/communication logs.
16. Serious adverse event (SAE) reports; IND Safety Reports.
17. Application to the IRB and approval for continuation of the protocol beyond the initial approval period.
18. Minutes and reports by Data Safety Monitoring Boards, if applicable.

7.A.4 INTERACTION BETWEEN THE QA SPECIALIST, THE INVESTIGATOR, AND THE STUDY TEAM

From an investigator's point of view, the most important part of the IRB's QA review—and the core of the QA program's educational objective—is the opportunity to review and discuss the QA specialist's findings, presented in a report. In some organizations, QA specialists prepare a preliminary report detailing any findings, and forward this to the investigator and study team members for comment. The investigator's review of the preliminary draft report provides an opportunity for the investigator to assess any deficiencies noted in the report, to point out—when appropriate—an incorrect finding, and discuss any recommendations contained in the report. The discussions between an investigator and the QA specialist is the most important element in the educational program embedded in the QA review. Investigators should not delegate the discussion to members of the study team, but should involve the study team in the discussions to enhance the educational effect of the QA process.

A review of the report allows investigators and members of the study team to explain issues that surfaced during the audit, understand what may be required for remedial action, and the possible need for additional training programs. Following review of the preliminary draft report, the QA specialist's final report is sent to the investigator and to the study team; some centers may incorporate the investigator's comments and/or plans for correcting deficiencies. The final report is generally sent to the chair of the IRB for review, but may also be distributed to a QA subcommittee of the IRB. A summary of the final report or full report may be presented to the full IRB at a regularly scheduled meeting per the QA program's SOP. On occasion, the report may be so poor that it leads to suspension or termination of a project. The IRB may rescind its approval of other ongoing research projects being performed by that investigator until issues of noncompliance have been satisfactorily resolved. Additionally, the IRB may refer the matter to institutional officials. Investigators may then be subject to scientific misconduct proceedings. The major focus of the QA audit should be the education of the investigators and their research teams.

A positive QA audit process, conducted under an organized and fully transparent process has the potential for providing highly focused and specific education on GCPs to investigators and study staff. It is an important tool for IRBs to demonstrate a commitment to protect subjects and the quality of clinical investigations. The QA process has enormous potential for heightening the awareness of investigators and study team members, when quality clinical investigations internalize GCPs into day-to-day performance of the study.

7.A.5 TAKE AWAY MESSAGES

- Investigators and IRBs benefit from a QA review—deficiencies can be corrected earlier in the process.
- Routine auditing by IRBs is becoming more widespread and a scheduled audit should not imply that there is anything wrong at the site.
- Trials with unusually high enrollments, involvement of potentially vulnerable populations, and inexperienced or previously non-compliant investigators should be considered for QA review.
- IRB QA programs should have written SOPs that should be shared with the investigators prior to beginning the review.
- Auditors may monitor the consent process and/or review patients' charts and essential documents.

NOTES

1. Announcement, Office of Human Research Protection (OHRP) Division of Assurances and Quality Improvement, Quality Improvement Program, 15 April 2002, *http://www.hhs.gov/ohrp/humansubjects/qip/qipdesc.pdf*, accessed 10 July 2004.

2. FDA Warning Letters, *http://www.fda.gov/foi/warning.htm*, accessed 10 July 2004; OHRP Determination Letters, *http://www.hhs.gov/ohrp/compliance/letters/index.html*, accessed 10 July 2004.

3. President's Commission for the Study of Ethical Problems in Medical and Biomedical and Behavioral Research, *Implementing Human Research Regulations: Second Biennial Report in the Adequacy and Uniformity of Federal Rules and Policies, and of their Implementation for the Protection of Human Subjects* (Washington, D.C.: U.S. Government Printing Office, 1983), 135-7; National Bioethics Advisory Commission, *Ethical and Policy Issues in Research Involving Human Participants* (Bethesda, Md.: NBAC, August 2001), 3; "Institutional Review Boards: Report and Recommendations of the National Commission for the Protection of Human Subjects of Biomedical and Behavioral Research," 43

Federal Register, 10 November 1978, p. 56174; *Scientific Research: Continued Vigilance Critical to Protecting Human Subjects* (Washington, D.C.: U.S. General Accounting Office, GAO/HEHS-96-72, March 1996), 17-8; DHHS Office of the Inspector General, *Institutional Review Boards: Their Role in Reviewing Approved Research* (Washington, D.C.: U.S. DHHS, OEI- 01-97-00190, June 1998), 7-8; DHHS Office of the Inspector General, *Institutional Review Boards: A Time for Reform* (Washington, D.C.: DHHS, OEI-01-97-00193, June 1998), 6-7; DHHS Office of the Inspector General, *Protecting Human Research Subjects: Status of Recommendations* (Washington, D.C.: DHHS, OEI-01-97-00197, April 2000), 2.

4. OHRP Determination Letters, *http://www.hhs.gov/ohrp/compliance/letters/index.html*, accessed 10 July 2004.

5. DHHS: 45 *CFR* 46.109; FDA 21 *CFR* 56.108; ICH Harmonized Tripartite Guideline, "Guideline for Good Clinical Practice E6," (recommended for adoption on 1 May 1996 by the ICH Steering Committee), *http://www.ich.org/pdfICH/e6.pdf*, accessed 6 June 2002.

6. "Guideline for Good Clinical Practice E6," ibid.

Part B: Inspections

Eileen Hilton, MD

What should the investigator, IRB, and sponsor expect when a regulatory agency inspects the organization or the investigator? These items will be considered in this section:

7.B.1 GENERAL CONSIDERATIONS OF REGULATORY AUTHORITY INSPECTIONS

Governmental regulators may inspect for a number of reasons, including, but not limited to, assuring the integrity of the clinical trial, validating data, and assuring the rights and safety of the enrolled subjects.

The Focus of the Inspections May Differ

Inspections of IRBs are now routinely performed (the FDA usually visits IRBs every three years or so). Alternatively, a clinical investigator may be the focus. Sponsors may inspect to review the records of clinical investigations. Although they are not specifically the focus of this book, manufacturing plants, sponsors, and CROs may be inspected as well.

What Triggers an Inspection

Audits may be performed routinely without any particular reason precipitating the inspection. The FDA performs such inspections at several hundred sites per year. A particular trial may be chosen for a study-focused audit when the investigation is "high profile," or it is considered pivotal. In these routine audits, sites that enroll the highest number of patients are the ones that are usually selected for inspection.

An investigator may be singled out for a nonroutine or "for cause" audit for a number of different reasons. Some investigators do an unusually large number of clinical trials, and this may arouse concern that they may be unable to manage so many studies without sacrificing personal oversight of each process. Other flags that initiate an audit are investigators who perform trials in areas that are outside of their field of specialization. Also suspect are suspiciously good data from studies that have a large number of enrollments, or "perfect" subject information that is inconsistent with data that has been reported at other sites that are performing the same trial.

"For cause" audits also occur in response to complaints or questions raised about the conduct of a trial. These complaints may be registered by a participant, a special interest group, or, not infrequently, by a member of the investigative team.

What Happens During the Inspection Process?

Notice of Inspection

In the case of an FDA inspection, a Form 482—Notice of Inspection will be sent to the principal investigator. The FDA may also call to schedule the audit. The site is usually given about a week's notice, but occasionally only a few days are given. It is prudent to notify all of those involved in a trial at the organization, including the IRB and pharmacy and laboratory personnel, when appropriate. If there is an industry sponsor, it should be notified as well. The FDA is not obliged to inform the sponsor of a site audit; however, the sponsor may be alerted to a potential inspection when it is queried about particular investigative sites. Many organizations have developed standard operating procedures (SOPs) that describe the management of a federal inspection. These usually include appointing an individual who will accompany the inspector throughout the process. SOPs usually address affidavits, photographs, and copies of source documents.

Preparation for an Inspection

The site should collect and have ready all necessary documents for the inspectors. The necessary information is the same as the essential documents listed in part 7.A.3 of this chapter. The auditors should be located in a comfortable place to review materials, close to a photocopy machine. The investigator and study or IRB staff should be available to answer any questions that may arise.

During the inspection, the following items will be examined: the roles and responsibilities of team members, the degree and appropriateness of delegation, where the study was performed, how the data was recorded, IRB review and the process of informed consent, investigational drug accountability, adherence to the protocol, safety reporting and compliance with local operating procedures, GCP, and other regulatory guidelines.

The inspector may review the study-related IRB files to ensure that IRB approval was obtained. The date of IRB approval will be verified. If there were adverse events, the inspector will ascertain if they were appropriately reported to the IRB. The inspector may ask to see the IRB's SOPs on adverse event reporting requirements for the organization. The inspector will look for protocol changes and how they were documented. Continuing review information will also be verified.

What Is a Form 483 and What Does it Mean?

The FDA Form 483 or List of Inspectional Observations is prepared by the inspector during the inspection visit; it will list findings of noncompliance. For the inspectee, the goal is to avoid receiving a Form 483. Once an item appears on a Form 483, it becomes part of the official record and is publicly available under the Freedom of Information Act (FOIA). Often, questions or issues that arise during the inspection can be addressed satisfactorily before they are entered onto the Form 483. But this can only happen if the research staff is readily available to respond to the investigator's questions.

Once the inspector is finished, an exit interview takes place and findings are discussed with involved parties. It is advisable to address the written findings that appear on the Form 483 in writing as soon as possible after the inspection. The written response should be nonadversarial and include: a confirmation of items corrected immediately, a description of actions to be taken and a timetable for correcting items not corrected immediately.

What Happens Next?

An Establishment Inspection Report (EIR) is prepared by the inspector for the FDA. This includes observations and discussions. The EIR is more detailed than the Form 483. It becomes part of the FDA's file on the facility and is available under the Freedom of Information Act. This may be used by sponsors to evaluate potential research sites. The FDA can follow up their findings with either judicial or nonjudicial remedies if indicated. There are several types of follow-up letters that may be issued, which include the following:

- NAI—No action indicated. This is an acknowledgment letter; it is the best kind to receive.
- VAI—Voluntary action indicated. This information letter is issued most frequently and should be addressed by the site.
- OAI—Official action indicated. Warning letter or invitation to informal conference; this is an unwelcome piece of mail. All issues cited should be addressed immediately and submitted in writing. The consequences of not taking this seriously can be ominous.

7.B.2 WHAT ARE THE MOST COMMON DEFICIENCIES REPORTED DURING CLINICAL INVESTIGATOR INSPECTIONS?

Listed in order of frequency, the most common deficiencies reported are:

- Protocol nonadherence,
- Inadequate/inaccurate records,
- IRB problems, including problems with submission of adverse events,
- Inadequate drug accountability,
- Problems with consent,
- Unapproved concomitant therapy.[1]

IRB Audits—When the IRB Is the Focus of an Audit

The most common IRB deficiencies cited after inspection are, in order of frequency:

- Failure to meet or maintain quorum,
- Inadequate or missing meeting minutes,
- Failure to maintain updated standard operating procedures,

- Poor record keeping,
- Roster problems—missing representation from certain specialties.[2]

7.B.3 BIOMEDICAL RESEARCH FRAUD

What is fraud in biomedical research? The federal definition is: "fabrication, falsification, or plagiarism in proposing, performing, or reviewing research, or in reporting research results." It is important to note that "research misconduct does not include honest error or differences of opinion."[3]

There are several well-publicized cases of biomedical fraud. One example occurred in 1998 when an investigator falsified data on multiple trials. Some of the acts included substitution of blood and urine samples from staff members for study subject's specimens. Further, study dropouts were replaced by another subject with the identity falsified. This case gave rise to criminal charges.[4] Subsequently, this investigator and three of his study coordinators were disbarred from doing research.

Detecting fraud in biomedical research is challenging. An experienced auditor uses on several clues. What arouses suspicion? Red flags occur when there are unusual attempts to delay an inspection. Other hints are difficulties obtaining source data from the study staff, and the atypical investigator who does all of the work alone. Another signal is blame shifting. Does the investigator try to place the blame on others?[5] Additional clues to detect fraud include:

- Everything is perfect. No mistakes are noted.
- All subjects completed the trial per protocol.
- Narrow range of laboratory readings.
- Suspiciously similar handwriting in subject's signature line and primary source documents.
- Similar lab values and subject characteristics.
- There are no subject errors on the diary cards.
- Several subjects with similar handwriting.
- Dates are inconsistent.
- Notes to the primary source that appear to be added after the original data.

Also, does the site's enrollment reflect a unique population or unusual results as compared to other sites performing the same trial? If so, do these subjects really exist? Incredibly, there have been reports of investigators creating fictitious subjects to fill enrollment. If the subjects exist, do they have the disease under study?

Possible Consequences

Chapter 1 detailed some of the measures that regulatory agencies may apply. To reiterate: an agency may disqualify the investigator and/or the data, or may suspend or terminate the clinical investigation. The FDA may also disqualify or suspend the clinical investigator if there has been repeated or deliberate failure to comply with applicable regulatory requirements or the clinical investigator has submitted false information to the sponsor or, if applicable, to the FDA. A disqualified clinical investigator cannot receive investigational drugs, biologics, or devices.

What Are Some of the Reasons for Disqualification?

- Repeated or deliberate submission of false data to the sponsor and FDA (21 *CFR* 312.70).
- Failure to obtain IRB approval and comply with IRB regulation (21 *CFR* 56).
- Failure to obtain informed consent (21 *CFR* 50).

- Failure to sign 1572 (21 *CFR* 312.60).
- Failure to follow the protocol (21 *CFR* 312.60).
- Failure to administer drugs under Principal Investigator supervision (21 *CFR* 312.61).
- Inadequate record keeping (21 *CFR* 312.62).
- Refusal to allow inspection of records (21 *CFR* 312.68).

The FDA publishes the names of clinical investigators who have been disqualified or "totally restricted."[6] Similarly to the FDA, OHRP makes its determinations public on its website.[7] These lists should be checked by sponsors and IRBs when an investigator applies for approval of a research project.

The government may decide to litigate. Although it is unusual, the criminal provisions of the Food and Drug Act can be applied to clinical investigators and IRB members. In the case cited previously for fraud, the investigator was fined $800,000 and sentenced to serve 15 months in federal prison.[8] How often do disciplinary actions occur? From 1964 through 1999, there were 99 disqualifications, 26 restrictions or actions with assurances, and 20 criminal prosecutions.[9]

THE IRB INSPECTION

What about inspections of IRBs? What types of problems evoke official action, and what might those actions entail? The problems that most often lead to official action include:

- Failure to prepare and/or follow written procedures
- Poor documentation
- Inadequate continuing review
- Inadequate fulfillment of requirements for expedited review
- Inadequate informed consent documents.[10]

7.B.4 WHAT ARE THE OFFICIAL ACTIONS THAT MAY RESULT FROM AN IRB AUDIT?

If OHRP is the regulator, it may restrict or withdraw its approval of an institution's assurance. There have been several high-profile examples involving institutions that have had to suspend all human research after an OHRP action.[11]

In the case of an FDA audit, if an IRB fails to respond adequately to allegations of noncompliance, the FDA may move to disqualify the IRB. Notice of disqualification will be sent to all parties, including the IRB of record, sponsors, and clinical investigators.[12]

In summary, any inspection or audit should be managed with a team approach—sponsor, IRB, and investigator should work together to provide the inspector with the appropriate information. Any issues, concerns, or deficiencies should be addressed and or corrected promptly and thoroughly in a nonadversarial manner.

7.B.5 TAKE AWAY MESSAGES

- Use published data such as FDA warning letters and OHRP determination letters to keep up to date on what may be required at an inspection.
- Notify all involved in the trial as soon as you are aware of a potential inspection.
- Appoint an individual who will accompany the inspector throughout the process.
- Research fraud is "fabrication, falsification, or plagiarism in proposing, performing, or reviewing research, or in reporting research results."
- "Research misconduct does not include

honest error or differences of opinion."

- An inspection of the investigative site may prompt subsequent inspections of the sponsor, clinical research organization (CRO) or site management organization (SMO), and the IRB.

NOTES

1. OHRP, Compliance Activities Common Findings and Guidance: *ohrp.osophs.dhhs.gov/references/findings.pdf*, accessed 12 July 2002; Clinical Investigator Deficiencies, FDA, *http://www.fda.gov/cder/present/dia-62000/woolen1/sld009.htm*, accessed 14 July 2002; Clinical Investigator Deficiency Categories, 1999, *http://www.fda.gov/cder/present/dia-62000/woolen1/sld008.htm*, accessed 14 July 2002.
2. IRB deficiencies: *http://www.fda.gov/cder/present/dia-62000/woolen1/sld015.htm*, accessed 14 July 2002.
3. Federal policy on research misconduct: *http://www.ostp.gov/html/001207_3.html*, accessed 16 July 2002.
4. *Fiddes* case background: *http://www.fda.gov/cder/present/dia-62000/woolen1/sld026.htm*, accessed 15 July 2002.
5. Tip for detection of serious misconduct: *http://www.fda.gov/cder/present/dia-62000/woolen1/sld043.htm*, accessed 14 July 2002.
6. FDA, Office of Regulatory Affairs, compliance references: bioresearch monitoring, *http://www.fda.gov/ora/compliance_ref/bimo/dis_res_assur.htm*, accessed 20 April 2002.
7. OHRP determination letters: *http://ohrp.osophs.dhhs.gov/detrm_letrs/lindex.htm*, accessed 14 July 2002.
8. *Fiddes*, see note 4 above.
9. Inspection outcomes: *http://www.fda.gov/cder/present/dia-62000/woolen1/sld011.htm*, accessed 14 July 2002.
10. Drug Information Association presentation by the FDA, June 2000, *http://www.fda.gov/cder/present/dia-62000/woolen1/sld016.htm*, accessed 15 July 2002.
11. Ethical violations and investigations: *http://www.researchprotection .org/govInvestigations.htm*, accessed 15 July 2002.
12. Disqualification of an IRB or institution: *http://www.fda.gov/oc/ohrt/irbs/appendixc.html*, accessed 15 July 2002.

8

Especially for IRB Staff

Elaine V. Neal, CIP, Victor W. Sidel, MD, Lillian Oshva, MD, Linda Reuter, MS, CIP, Kendra Dimond, Esq., Mary R. Marta, Esq., and Philip Mitchell, Esq.

This chapter offers general guidance and practical advice to IRB administrators, IRB members, and institutional officials. It also delves into legal, conflict-of-interest, and insurance liability issues confronting organizations that conduct research involving human subjects.

Chapter 8 is comprised of the following parts:

Part A: IRB Management

Elaine V. Neal, CIP

8.A.1 A PRIMER FOR IRB ADMINISTRATORS

The direction, management, and oversight of all activities and staff relative to the effective administration and function of an IRB and human subjects research program can seem to be an extremely demanding duty. But, more often, it is a responsibility that offers subtle and unseen rewards, for example:

- A progress report from an investigator indicates that cancer subjects who have been refractory to other treatments are responding well to the study drug, with minimal side-effects and improved quality of life.
- A phone call from a new coordinator who wants to thank you for helping her through her first protocol submission to the IRB.
- The looks on the faces of the new fellows as they watch a presentation on the realities and horrors of Nazi experimentation.

These are just a few of the reasons that IRB administrators choose to enter and remain in their chosen profession. What we do and how we do it isn't quite as important as *why*, but the *what* and *how* help us to satisfy the *why*. The range and scope of IRB administrators' responsibilities are varied, complex, and broad. Although an IRB administrator's duties may differ slightly from IRB to IRB, the following is a relatively comprehensive delineation.

- Provide leadership and increase the IRB's efficiency and quality of functioning in support of the research program; protect human subjects by improving compliance, increasing resources, and performing continuous quality improvement.
- Direct the activities of the IRB to maintain a high level of quality in its administration through careful fiscal and facilities management.
- Evaluate existing procedures and policies and develop and implement revised policies and procedures in accordance with all applicable federal, state, local, and institutional requirements.
- Identify and assess problematic issues and institute effective resolution.
- Provide counsel and expertise to investigators, coordinators, staff, and IRB members on the appropriate conduct of research and preparation of protocol and consent documents in accordance with all applicable federal, state, and local regulations and the International Conference on Harmonisation (ICH) *Good Clinical Practice Guidelines*[1] and standard operating procedures.
- Represent the IRB and the organization in communications with federal, state, and local authorities.
- Provide expertise to other segments of the organization on issues that may influence the conduct of research.
- Manage/oversee all activities related to IRB meetings, including but not limited to the following:
    - Pre-administrative tasks such as performing preliminary review of agenda items (for example, new submissions, modifications), assigning reviewers, distributing meeting materials, and communicating with investigators and reviewers to address any concerns or questions.
    - Post-meeting administrative tasks such as preparation of minutes and communicating decisions to investigators.
- Assure the appropriate review and monitoring of all research activities.
- Review, investigate, and report on allegations of noncompliance and supervise implementation of resolution and remediation.
- Oversee the development and implementation of education and training programs for IRB staff, research investigators, IRB members, and the lay community.

- Develop and maintain a nonadversarial culture of respect for compliance that promotes a sense of partnership.

It is important to note that not all IRB administrators share the same responsibilities. At some institutions, an IRB administrator's responsibilities encompass a broad range of duties like those described above. It is in these organizations that an IRB administrators is perceived as an authority on compliance and oversight. The administrator's role is professional, with responsibility for all aspects of the IRB process and its related procedures. Other institutions view IRB administrators more as administrative assistants who have a limited range of duties that are focused primarily on procedure.[2] The former is preferable as well as practical, as IRB administrators function as comprehensive professionals on whom the organization can rely for leadership and compliance/regulatory expertise, in addition to overseeing the management of the IRB.

IRBs are charged with protecting human subjects in the research studies they oversee.[3] IRB administrators provide the leadership and guidance necessary to manage all of the activities and staff related to this. IRB administrators are comprehensive professionals who are leaders, authority figures, and counselors who are responsible for "the Five Ps"—people, processes, procedures, policies, and problems.

8.A.2 RELATIONSHIPS

One of the most important components of IRB administrators' responsibilities is to maintain good relationships with the IRB chair, the IRB staff and membership, the investigators, and the coordinators—it is through these relationships that an IRB successfully carries out its function: the protection of human research subjects.

Interaction with IRB Chairs

The relationship between IRB administrators and IRB chairs is perhaps the most important with respect to its effect on the form and function of an IRB. IRB administrators and IRB chairs are the leadership team that guide and direct an IRB.[4] Open and direct communication—in addition to mutual respect—must exist to create and sustain an effective and efficient IRB. IRB administrators and IRB chairs support each other, and each has unique expertise.

IRB administrators and IRB chairs work together toward the common goal of protecting research subjects while they maintain the integrity of the research effort through the proficiency of their IRB. Administrators should meet regularly with IRB chairs to outline specific objectives and concerns and to discuss other issues or responsibilities that are essential to the successful management of the IRB.

Interaction with IRB Staff

Another important relationship exists between IRB administrators and their staffs. IRB administrators must be able to communicate effectively to cultivate a successful team. To this end, frequent staff meetings should be held. Such meetings provide a forum for continuing education of staff, wherein new information is disseminated and creative ideas are encouraged. When IRB administrators promote teamwork, accountability, and creativity, they help other IRB professionals to work together to achieve a common goal. Capable IRB administrators develop and maintain a knowledgeable, cohesive, and committed staff, and create an environment in which the protection of human subjects is the prime directive.

Interaction with Investigators

IRB administrators must represent the best interest of research subjects while they maintain the integrity of the research effort. To accomplish this, administrators must encourage open communication between investigators and the IRB as well as a sense of mutual respect and cooperation.[5] The relationship between the IRB and investigators can sometimes be tenuous; some investigators view IRBs as bureaucratic impediments to research. Others have—through the efforts of the IRB leadership and high-level institutional support—learned that the IRB is an important partner in the research process. It is difficult to promote the importance and authority of the IRB in an organization in which high-level support is lacking.

IRB administrators should foster a congenial relationship between the IRB and investigators. This can be accomplished through open and honest communication. It is important that investigators understand the rationale behind what the IRB does and expects. Discussions with investigators should include explanations of the basis for the IRB's decisions and the purposes of its policies. It is also important to provide guidance and make recommendations on how investigators might better communicate and work with the IRB. Relationships between investigators and the IRB are vital to any research program. Investigators must be reminded that IRB administrators and the IRB committee protect research subjects as well as the integrity of the research program. It is through compliance that both objectives are met.

Although the prime directive of every IRB is the protection of human research subjects, and this must take precedence over all other concerns, it is also essential to promote the ethical and appropriate conduct of research to protect the integrity of the research program.

Interaction with Sponsors

Recent discussions within the IRB community[6] indicate that most IRB administrators prefer not to communicate directly with sponsors. Other administrators, however, believe that some interaction is necessary to expedite the review and approval process. In any case, it is important to note that an IRB's relationship is with investigators, not with sponsors. IRB staff should not act as an extension of investigators' staff, nor should they provide services to sponsors' representatives.

Some matters may be more easily resolved by direct communication with sponsors' representatives, specifically when there is question regarding what regulations state versus what sponsors may "demand." Although this author maintains a policy of communicating only with investigators, an occasional phone call or e-mail directly to a sponsor to clarify an issue can reduce possible miscommunication among all of the parties involved and expedite the process.

Interactions with the Membership

The relationship between the IRB membership and an IRB administrator should be one of mutual respect. The relationship is akin to that previously outlined in the discussion on the relationship with investigators, in that it is important to create a sense of camaraderie, cooperation, and unity by direct communication and education. IRB administrators should encourage active participation and understanding of the function and processes of the IRB in its membership. Members should be encouraged to discuss issues and concerns with their IRB administrator or chair. This will significantly contribute to the overall success of the IRB.

It is also essential that a connection between an IRB and the local research community exist. Very often members of an IRB are also investigators, and it is their appreciation of the operational process as well as the practical aspects of research that facilitate the sharing of information and that can enhance knowledge and efficacy among the membership.

Unfortunately, some IRB members who are colleagues or subordinates of an investigator may feel coerced or intimidated in carrying out their dual roles. Although the identities of reviewers should be kept confidential, this does not always happen. It is therefore imperative that IRB members who find themselves in this position be supported and shielded as much as is possible. The IRB c(air may need to intervene and act as an intermediary between the parties to resolve difficulties that may arise.

8.A.3 MANAGING THE PAPERS WHILE PROTECTING THE SUBJECTS

All too often IRBs are viewed as creating bureaucratic obstacles. Although IRBs seek to facilitate research efforts, it is easy to see why investigators might not believe that to be the case, given the number of forms they are often required to submit for review of their proposals. In addition to forms for new submissions, there are often forms and documentation required for continuing review, adverse events, modifications, et cetera. When multiplied by "x" number of investigators and protocols, the management of this tremendous volume of paperwork is an arduous task for IRB administrators and their staffs. Add to this the additional large number of other miscellaneous administrative documents required, and the requirements may seem to be overwhelming. What can IRB administrators do?

- Be organized. Pay attention to detail.
- Develop internal processes to streamline the workload. Re-evaluate periodically.
- Be aware of what each member of your staff is working on at any given time.
- Solicit ideas from staff and other research professionals on how to improve a process.
- Know when to ask for help and recognize when a member of your staff needs help.
- Make "to-do" lists—stick to them.
- Prioritize, delegate/disseminate, act, follow through, and follow up.
- Develop and maintain, or purchase a computerized database management system to monitor and manage the research program.

There are a number of reasonably priced, commercially available, fully integrated, IRB-specific software packages that track protocols and provide continuing review, monitor adverse events, as well as prepare pre- and post-meeting documents. A comprehensive database management system is essential, as it can help to manage and monitor all research activities, and so strengthen compliance and streamline IRB functions and processes.

Although every IRB office may not always be fully staffed, the increase in federal audits, suspensions of research, and local quality improvement initiatives in recent years make it unlikely that severe understaffing will be able to continue for any length of time. These monitoring activities have led to increases in the staffing and resources available to many IRBs. Depending on the volume of research they handle, it is feasible that most IRB offices will include, at minimum, the following staff.

- One director/administrator,
- One or two senior-level staff persons,
- Two additional staff persons.

This example is based on an IRB that meets once monthly, reviews approximately 300 new protocols per year, and whose portfolio consists of approximately 1,000 active research studies. IRBs that review fewer protocols and meet less frequently will not require the same level of staffing.

Each of these staff persons should have specific, assigned tasks. IRB administrators should monitor the flow of paperwork, avoiding bottlenecks. This can be achieved by ensuring that each staff person prioritizes, delegates, and acts promptly on every piece of paper that crosses their desks. It is imperative that follow through and follow up be performed in a timely manner in order to avoid unnecessary delay.

By prioritizing, directing, acting, and following up on paperwork in a timely manner, it is possible to manage the volume of paperwork so that attention can be paid to the more important responsibility of protecting the individuals who agree to participate in research.

8.A.4 PROCESSES, PROCEDURES, POLICIES, AND PROBLEMS

The role of IRB administrators has evolved significantly in response to increased oversight responsibilities and enhanced surveillance by federal agencies. What at one time might have been a secretarial or lower-level administrative function has become a high-level professional position in most large organizations. IRB administrators oversee daily operational issues and concerns, including the administration of the office and all activities related to the function of the IRB. Management and development of human resources is critically important, and the efficiency and effectiveness of an IRB depends on its processes. Therefore, quality improvement activities should be initiated to identify areas that may require enhancement or expansion. Once a quality improvement program is implemented, quality improvement/quality assurance must continue. The Department of Health and Human Services (DHHS) Office for Human Research Protections (OHRP) recently launched a quality improvement program to help IRBs evaluate and improve the quality of their human research protection programs. OHRP will collaborate with IRBs and others within the research community (subjects, institutions, investigators, sponsors, the public) to improve the human subjects' protection system.[7] This initiative provides IRBs with the support needed to enhance their individual research programs and concentrate on protecting subjects.

As a result of their expertise, IRB administrators are seen as regulatory authorities and resources on questions regarding policy and compliance. IRB administrators understand the practical aspects of the review process, the conduct of research, and how to apply ethical and regulatory standards. To achieve such proficiency, successful IRB administrators must stay current with regulations that apply to the appropriate review and ethical conduct of research. Such regulations are promulgated by the DHHS (45 *CFR* 46)[8] and the Food and Drug Administration (FDA) (21 *CFR* 50, 56, 312, 812).[9] Other agency regulations may apply in certain situations. State and international regulations may also apply (for example, the ICH *Good Clinical Practice Guidelines*.)[10] The ethical principles and guidelines on which these regulations were based include *The Belmont Report*,[11] the World Medical Association's *Declaration of Helsinki*,[12] and *The Nuremberg Code*.[13] Regulations may require review when agencies issue new guidance.

Compliance Oversight

Issues of noncompliance are the most unpleasant concerns that IRB administrators may confront. Incidents of noncompliance must be formally reviewed, investigated, and reported to the appropriate authorities (for example, DHHS OHRP, FDA, funding agencies, et cetera). Resolution and remediation must be prompt. These activities are usually conducted by IRB administrators in consultation with IRB chairs, legal counsel, and/or a compliance or regulatory officer, in addition to the IRB committee. Investigations into noncompliance may be conducted through the use of an ad hoc committee, a special subcommittee of the IRB, in addition to the involvement of IRB administrators and IRB chair. Such investigations are brought to the full committee for their information and/or recommendation.

In situations when the IRB or IRB office is found to be noncompliant or remiss in its responsibilities (perhaps as a result of an OHRP or FDA audit), it is imperative that the IRB address the event in a similar manner and immediately institute measures to prevent reoccurrence.

As a result of efforts on the federal level to foster a more friendly, interactive federal-IRB relationship and to promote a better understanding of the regulations and their applicability in the IRB setting (specifically, recent initiatives by OHRP), educational programs are being established at institutions throughout the IRB community that will contribute greatly to investigators' and IRBs' awareness of the appropriate conduct of research.

8.A.5 THE IRB ADMINISTRATOR AS A VOTING MEMBER OF THE IRB

There is disagreement among IRB professionals on whether IRB administrators should serve as voting members of an IRB.[14] Advocates believe that IRB administrators should serve as voting members because of the expertise they bring to the committee. This expertise is invaluable when deliberating on protocols. Their inclusion may also promote respect for IRB administrators and their authority and credibility. Further, IRB administrators must be voting members of their IRB to conduct expedited or exempt review (or participate in continuing review).[15]

Other IRB professionals disagree and argue that IRB administrators should not serve as voting members because they are often called to assist in the preparation of research proposals, and therefore could be considered advocates of the research. It is further argued that when IRB administrators maintain distance from the IRB, it provides them with time to administer to a more service-oriented office.

8.A.6 CONTINUING EDUCATION IS A MUST

IRB administrators should promote and provide continuing education to staff, IRB members, and investigators. Through their knowledge of the specific requirements, as set forth by oversight agencies, IRB administrators can foster credibility, as well as respect, for the sometimes onerous mission of overseeing a research program.

Administrators can further their knowledge and obtain information on new and emerging issues, regulations, and requirements by attending professional conferences and continuing education programs. It is important to participate in presentations and workshops that address or discuss concerns relevant to the protection of human subjects and the research environment. In addition, memberships in professional societies such as the Applied Research Ethics National Association (ARENA), the Society of Research administrators (SRA), the Society of Clinical Research Associates (SoCRA), the Association of Clinical Research Professionals (ACRP), and so on, offer other ways to interact with colleagues and enhance our understanding of new and emerging requirements and trends. Administrators can maintain a progressive knowledge base through the use of professional journals and publications, internet web sites, federal and professional internet listservs, and the media at large. Chapter 6 of this book and "Useful Websites," at the end of the book, offer additional information on continuing education.

Continuing education is imperative to ensure compliance and increase awareness in the research community. It is increasingly obvious that the general public benefits from aggressive educational campaigns. Media attention to recent incidents of noncompliance with ethical and regulatory standards has led to increased scrutiny of IRBs. Aggressive campaigns can increase awareness regarding research involving human subjects and stimulate a positive attitude toward this research. IRB administrators should implement educational initiatives to achieve these objectives.

8.A.7 TAKE AWAY MESSAGES

IRB administrators' responsibilities encompass the direction, management, and oversight of all activities and staff relative to the administration and function of IRBs. The chief responsibility of an administrator is to protect research subjects. This is achieved in part by leading through example. The protection of human subjects in research is our prime directive!

- "The Five Ps"
  - *People:* leadership, direction, motivation
  - *Processes:* evaluate, implement, improve
  - *Procedures:* review, institute, enhance
  - *Policies:* interpret, apply, re-evaluate
  - *Problems:* identify, assess, resolve
- Prioritize, delegate, act, follow through, and follow up.
- Communicate effectively and professionally.
- Educate investigators, IRB members, and staff on the rationale for IRB policy.
- Encourage information and idea sharing. Be open to new ideas.
- Continuing education for everyone!
- Develop and maintain a culture of respect and compliance. Avoid adversarial interaction.
- Implement a quality improvement program and perform continuous quality improvement to maintain a successful and streamlined IRB process.

NOTES

1. ICH, *Good Clinical Practical Guidelines*, 1996, *http://www.ifpma.org/ich5e.html.*

2. E. Bankert and R. Amdur, *IRB Management and Function: The IRB Administrative Director* (Sudbury, Mass.: Jones & Bartlett, 2002).

3. 21 *CFR* 50 Subpart B and 21 *CFR* 56.102, updated 1998, *http://www.fda.gov/oc/ohrt/irbs/appendixb. html* and *http://www.fda.gov/oc/ohrt/irbs/appendix c.html;* 45 *CFR* 46 Subpart A, revised 13 November 1997, *http://ohrp.osophs.dhhs.gov/human subjects/guidance/45cfr46.htm;* World Medical Association, "Basic Principles for All Medical Research" (paragraph 13), *Declaration of Helsinki*, adopted by the 18th WMA General Assembly Helsinki, Finland, June 1964 and amended by the 52nd WMA General Assembly, Edinburgh, Scotland, October 2000, *http://www.wma.net/e/policy/17-c_e.html.*

4. See note 2 above.

5. Ibid.
6. The IRB Discussion Forum, updated 10 July 2002, *http://www.irbforum.com,* accessed 26 June 2002.
7. Division of Assurances of Quality Improvement, Office for Human Research Protections, *http://ohrp.osophs.dhhs.gov/humansubjects/qip/qip.htm.*
8. 45 *CFR* 46, revised 13 November 1997, *http://ohrp.osophs.dhhs.gov/humansubjects/guidance/45cfr46.tym.*
9. 21 *CFR* 50, 56, 312, 812, updated 1998, *http://www.fda.gov/oc/ohrt/irbs/.*
10. See note 1 above.
11. Office of the Secretary, Ethical Principals and Guidelines for the Protection of Human Subjects of Research, the National Commission for the Protection of Human Subjects of Biomedical and Behavioral Research, *The Belmont Report,* updated 18 April 1979, *http://phrp. osophs.dhhs.goiv/humansubjects/guidance/belmont.htm.*
12. *Declaration of Helsinki,* see note 3 above.
13. *The Nuremberg Code, Trials of War Criminals before the Nuremberg Military Tribunals under Control Council Law No. 10,* vol. 2 (Washington, D.C.: U.S. Government Printing Office, 1949), 181-2.
14. See note 1 above.
15. 45 *CFR* 46.110 (revised 13 November 1997), *http://ohrp.osophs.dhhs.gov/humansubjects/guidance/45cfr46htm.*

Part B: The IRB Chairperson

Victor W. Sidel, MD

This section focuses on chairing an IRB.

8.B.1 THE ROLES OF THE IRB CHAIR

IRB chairs play an important role in the work of an IRB. They must in part be enthusiastic leaders; experts on legal and ethical issues and on federal, state, and local regulations governing research with human subjects and on governing IRBs; synthesizers; taskmasters; and diplomats. They must be enthusiastic leaders, because many members of IRBs find that the time consumed by IRB work interferes with other work they do. In this time of severe economic pressures on hospitals, medical practice, and researchers, IRB chairs must help inspire IRB members to perform their IRB work well. IRB chairs must be experts on the legal and ethical issues faced by IRBs and on the federal, state, and local regulations that govern human research and IRBs, because the complexities of the issues and regulations have increased dramatically in recent years. IRB chairs must be synthesizers, because the discursive discussions in many full IRB meetings demand clear and concise restatement if decisions are to be expeditiously made. IRB chairs must be taskmasters, because the rules, regulations, and deadlines that govern IRBs must be rigorously respected. Finally, chairs must be diplomats, because the interests of subjects, the community, investigators, and institutions demand full respect and appropriate mediation.

On the other hand, IRB chairs do not need to be experts on the scientific basis or on the benefits and risks of the protocols that their IRBs review. Other members of the IRB and others inside and outside the organization may be relied on to perform those expert roles. IRB chairs must help enlist the advice of these experts and should have a clear understanding of the information and advice provided by the experts, to help interpret that information and advise the members of the IRB. This requires extensive reading of materials published on issues of research involving human subjects and on informed consent, attending relevant conferences, and consulting with colleagues both within and outside the institution.

Although there are other important roles, the most important role of IRB chairs is protection of human subjects. An essential element in this protection is absolute protection of the right of potential subjects to refuse to enter into a research program, and of the right of enrolled subjects to withdraw from participation at any time. Protection of this "right to refuse" requires not only full appreciation of the right itself, but also full appreciation of ways to implement it. IRB chairs should keep in mind the words of Hans Jonas: "Let us all remember that a slower progress in the conquest of disease would not threaten society, grievous as it is to those who deplore that particular disease be not yet conquered, but that society would indeed be threatened by the erosion of those moral values whose loss, possibly caused by too ruthless a pursuit of scientific progress, would make its most dazzling triumphs not worth having."[1]

8.B.2 DUTIES TO SUBJECTS

Protecting Subjects' Right to Refuse

The right to refuse is associated, as most rights are, with a duty. To protect this right, it is the duty of the investigator to obtain valid informed consent from each subject.

The elements necessary for a valid informed consent, for either treatment or research, are generally considered to include:

- Threshold elements (preconditions):
  - Competence (legal standing to understand and to decide),
  - Capacity (cognitive ability to understand and to decide), and
  - Voluntariness (in making the decision).
- Information elements:
  - Disclosure (of relevant information),
  - Recommendation (of participation in a therapeutic intervention or in a research program), and
  - Understanding (of the disclosure and the recommendation).
- Consent elements:
  - Decision (in favor of participation) and
  - Authorization (of participation).[2]

IRB chairs have a duty to ensure that all of these elements are included in an informed consent process that has IRB approval, and to participate in developing and implementing methods for determining that the process is conducted properly. IRB chairs have responsibilities to ensure that the investigator honors the threshold elements and the consent elements; but the greatest attention must be given to the information elements: disclosure, recommendation, and understanding.

Disclosure

The investigator who seeks consent from the subject for participation in a research project has a duty to disclose the following:

1. The nature and the prognosis of the condition being studied,
2. The nature of the research,
3. The potential benefits and risks of the research,
4. The alternatives, including a refusal to participate in the research, and the potential consequences of each, and
5. The conflicts of interest a researcher may have in making the recommendation to the subject for participation in the research.[3]

1. The Nature and Prognosis of the Condition Being Studied

The underlying mindset of many clinicians when they seek consent for a clinical procedure is paternalistic. Clinicians assume the right to select information that they believe would provide benefit to patients and the right to suppress the revelation of information that would or would not be useful or would cause harm. Hippocrates' admonition is still followed by many clinicians today: "Perform [your duties] calmly and adroitly, concealing most things from the patient while you are attending to him. Give necessary orders with cheerfulness and serenity, turning his attention away from what is being done to him; sometimes reprove sharply and emphatically, and sometimes comfort with solicitude and attention, revealing nothing of the patient's future or present condition."[4] In short, according to this view, deception or coercion are not only ethically permissible, but may be encouraged in clinical practice when clinicians perceive them as helpful to patients. Clinicians at times will provide additional information to family or others caring for patients with the assumption that some of the information will be conveyed to patients at "an appropriate time." While many and possibly most clinicians would consider this practice ethical and beneficial, its legality is unclear.

Investigators have no such loopholes. The nature of the condition and the prognosis must be clearly disclosed. Deception and coercion of human subjects to induce participation in research, or reliance on family members to disclose relevant information at a later time are, with extremely rare exceptions, not ethically permissible and may be legally perilous.

2. The Nature of the Research

Clinicians may, in the "best interest of patients," wish to gloss over details of treatment or even lie about the nature of the treatment. Most clinicians these days would, to some extent, disagree with such an approach. But so long as the reasons for the deception are based on the principles of "beneficence" or "non-maleficence," and the clinical outcome is satisfactory, clinicians are unlikely to get into legal difficulties by failure to tell the whole truth.

Again, investigators have no such loopholes. The nature of research must, with rare exceptions, be clearly disclosed. The rare exceptions, which generally lie in the field of psychological or perception research, require that the obfuscation have a valid research purpose, that the obfuscation cause no lasting harm to the subjects, that investigators explain the obfuscation and the reason for it to the subjects at the end of the experiment, and that a review committee such as an IRB approve the research and the obfuscation. Otherwise it is generally accepted that investigators disclose to the subjects the truth, the whole truth, and nothing but the truth about the nature and the details of the research.

This includes disclosure, in language understandable to the subjects, of relevant details, such the nature of Phase I or Phase II clinical trials, randomized clinical trials, the use of placebos or of withholding of effective treatment, the blinding of study personnel, and other arcane matters. The fact that the study is being conducted at multiple sites should also be discussed, especially if an IRB at another site has rejected or modified the protocol.

Finally, some protocols are so complex and others are so hazardous that review bodies may permit only investigators or other knowledgeable members of the research team to volunteer for the study, although this of course involves the potential for coercion.

3. The Potential Benefits and Risks

For both treatment and research, the potential benefits and risks of the research protocol must be clearly disclosed. The potential problem here is usually not deception, but rather exaggeration of the potential benefits and minimization of the risks. Exaggeration of the expected benefits may be caused by the enthusiasm or the self-interest of the clinician or investigator. Exaggeration of benefits in obtaining consent for clinical treatment may not, in itself, be dysfunctional and may indeed, under special circumstances, be of benefit to the patient, but it is never acceptable in obtaining consent from subjects for participation in research.

Similarly, it is essential to disclose all of the elements of potential risk to patients or subjects—including physical, psychological, and social risks. The virtual impossibility of foreseeing all of the possible risks and of conveying clearly the known risks increase the dangers of minimization. Additional problems lie in the imprecision of knowledge of benefits and risks and in the imprecision of language with which to convey them. A "small" risk may mean, for example, that a very few patients or subjects may experience large problems, or that large numbers of patients or subjects may experience minor problems. The elements of disclosure, particularly for participation in research, must be as extensive, as precise, and as clear as possible. The elements must also be relevant to the decision to be made. Long lists of potential adverse reactions may have legal importance, but may be of less use to patients or subjects than a more focused discussion of the potential risks.

4. The Alternatives, Including a Refusal to Participate, and the Potential Consequences

For both treatment and research, the alternatives, including refusing to accept the recommended treatment or the offered participation in research, must be clearly disclosed. The potential problem here is usually not deception, but failure to include all the alternatives, minimization of the potential benefits of the alternatives, and exaggeration of the risks of the alternatives. The option to refuse the recommended treatment, or the option to refuse offered participation in research, or the option to participate in a more limited way, is not usually expressed as clearly as is the option of "acquiescence" in the recommendation.

5. Conflicts of Interest a Researcher May Have

The conflicts of interest clinicians or investigators have that may be important to patients' or subjects' understanding of the treatment or research, of the risks and benefits, of the alternatives, and—most important—of the recommendations, must be disclosed. Issues of conflict of interest are also discussed in chapter 5. There are many problems associated with "mixed agency"—the playing of more than one role or of "serving more than one master"—in modern medical practice. Clinicians in fee-for-service practice may benefit financially by doing more tests or providing more treatment; clinicians in managed-care practices may benefit financially by doing fewer tests or providing less treatment. Researchers may benefit financially, academically, in prestige and honor, or in other ways from their research. The department or the institution may bring considerable pressure on clinicians to treat patients in a particular way or may bring considerable pressure on investigators to initiate a research project or to recruit more subjects. Sponsors, particularly those that have a financial stake in the use of a treatment or in the outcome of research, may at times be relentless and uncritical in their advocacy.

The Recommendation for Participation

The recommendation, if one is made, must be crystal clear. The difference between a recommendation for treatment and for participation in research lies in the view that it is reasonable for patients to expect that a recommendation for a therapeutic intervention is made for their benefit; when consent for participation in a research program is requested, there is an underlying presumption of potential benefit to others. If subjects may also personally benefit from participation (in addition to the satisfaction of altruistic contribution to medical knowledge), that may be explained, but the explanation must make clear that the benefit is uncertain and that the constraints and additional tests that are usually part of a research protocol may be different than those involved in a treatment protocol.

Clinicians may wish, and perhaps should try, to persuade a patient to agree to a recommendation that they believe would best serve the patient's medical interests. Ultimately, however, clinicians must usually accede to the patient's decision, however "senseless" or "unreasonable" it may appear. Clinicians may choose to withdraw from further participation in a patient's care when this happens. Investigators, on the other hand, must permit subjects to make their own decisions on participation in research or withdrawal from it without undue persuasion. Recognition of the right to refuse and presumption of competence and capacity to refuse are even more important in seeking consent for research than in seeking consent for therapeutic intervention.

Understanding

Investigators and clinicians have a duty to assure patients' or subjects' understanding of the disclosure and the recommendation. The use of simple language and of interpreters and translated forms to assist comprehension when a patient or a subject's degree of literacy and/or knowledge of English are in question are relatively straightforward. Formal testing for comprehension may be difficult. While it is usually possible for clinicians or researchers to determine the degree of understanding of a patient or subject by using question-and-answer or other Socratic techniques, this is extremely difficult and few clinicians or researchers will take the time to do so. The application of such techniques by knowledgeable observers without a self-interest in the decision would certainly be preferable to evaluation of understanding by clinicians or investigators, but such procedures are difficult to establish. Again, understanding of risk and potential benefit by subjects is at least as important, and may be more important, than understanding by patients in a therapeutic situation. The IRB chair has an important part of the responsibility for instituting processes that ensure this understanding.

8.B.3 THE PROTECTION OF ESPECIALLY VULNERABLE SUBJECTS

The protection of the right of refusal of especially vulnerable subjects—pregnant women, fetuses, children, prisoners—is one of IRB chairs' most important responsibilities. Chairs must know the regulatory requirements for the protection of each of these groups and insist that they be rigorously followed.

Pregnant Women

Research that involves pregnant women may impose risks not only to the woman but also to the fetus. Since the fetus is obviously in no position itself to refuse to participate, the right of refusal on behalf of the welfare of the fetus is particularly important. The request for the informed consent of the woman must make clear not only the possible risks to her, but also the potential risks to her fetus. When the father is known and available, regulations may require that he too should be asked for informed consent to research that may harm the fetus. The chair must, in helping guide the IRB, attempt to balance protection of the right of refusal by the mother or the father for the benefit of the fetus against the right of the mother to accept research that has potential direct benefit to her.

Children

Research that involves children also requires special attention by IRB chairs. Although state laws differ, people younger than a statutory age determined by a state are not considered legally competent to consent formally to research. But many children nonetheless have "decisional capacity"; they can understand the nature of the research, their options, and the consequences of their decision. Chairs must help their IRB determine the nature of the right of minors to refuse to participate and how that can be protected in specific protocols under review by the IRB.

Prisoners

Research involving prisoners has raised special ethical issues, since prisoners are literally a "captive population." While on the one hand they may have full competence and capacity to understand and to consent to research, often they face other constraints: they may be under enormous pressure to consent to participate in the research in anticipation of special "credits" for parole or other benefits, such as needed medical treatment that might otherwise not be available.

8.B.4 PROCEDURES

IRB chairs must assume general oversight of the work of staff members who prepare materials for expedited reviews and for presentation at full meetings of the IRB, of the work of reviewers, and of the work of auditors of the research after it has been approved. This includes oversight of preparations for full meetings, such as the preparation of agendas and the assurance that a quorum will be present.

IRB chairs have the responsibility to issue approval and rejection letters and to issue letters that explain the reasons for deferral. While there is no requirement that chairs must personally sign such letters, they must designate the person or persons who have the authority to sign. This work, and the preparation of the minutes of each full IRB meeting, must be carefully overseen, but without interfering with the initiative of each staff member.

One of the most important tasks of chairs in chairing meetings of the full IRB is expediting the discussion and the decision making of the IRB so that its tasks can be completed in the allotted time. Equally important, however, is assuring that there is sufficient time for adequate discussion of risks to subjects. It has been my experience that if IRB meetings last more than two hours, the interest of the members begins to flag and the quality of the discussion and of the decisions of the IRB may begin to deteriorate.

8.B.5 DEALING WITH IRB MEMBERS, INVESTIGATORS, AND REVIEWERS

An extremely important part of the work of IRB chairs is maintaining the enthusiasm of IRB members. The IRB meetings should not only be informative but also exciting. IRB chairs have a responsibility to promote and to reflect this excitement.

An important and delicate task of IRB chairs is to deal with investigators who, because of ignorance or design, do not obey the rules for submitting, conducting, reporting, or renewing their studies. Similarly, reviewers who do not perform their duties adequately must be guided by chairs to perform them better, or replacements should be selected.

Some IRBs also have vice-chairs or deputy chairs. These roles are extremely important, and the individuals who serve in this capacity should be confident of the value and significance of their positions. The roles of each should be explicitly clear and should include ample opportunities for contributions to the work of the IRB.

8.B.6 THE "ART OF CHAIRING"

The competence, thoughtfulness, and commitment of the membership of an IRB are vital to the successful performance of its tasks. The IRB must deal with complex issues in depth and in ways that foster the protection of research subjects. Chairs must ensure the competence of IRB members and encourage seriousness with which they approach this important work. They must be able to look forward eagerly to each meeting. These meetings are opportunities to work with the staff of the IRB and with its members to help create an atmosphere in which the critically important work of the advancement of medical knowledge and improved care of patients will not compromise the rights or the safety of those who contribute to this work by acting as research subjects. Above all, IRB chairs must be sensitive to the feelings of other IRB members, the staff, and the administration.

The chair of the committee pays an important role by keeping the discussion focused and moving forward. Knowing when to bring issues to a vote, table particular discussions until more information becomes available, and consult with IRB resource personnel (IRB lawyer, staff member, et cetera) is most important. IRB chairs often craft compromises among group members, allowing for speedy solutions on which all members of the group can agree.

8.B.7 CHANGES IN THE ROLE OF IRBs AND THEIR CHAIRS

In 1968 colleagues and I at the Massachusetts General Hospital brought to the hospital's Research Committee (which also had responsibility to protect human subjects) a proposal to perform a randomized clinical trial involving patients who were admitted to the hospital with uncomplicated acute myocardial infarction (MI). The protocol called for randomization of patients on the fifth day of their hospitalization into two groups, who would have different lengths of stay, so long as no complications developed. The "control" group would have the standard length of stay for uncomplicated myocardial infarction at that time, a total of three weeks; the "experimental" group would have a length of stay shortened to a total of two weeks. At that time, there had been no randomized clinical trials comparing length of stay for patients with uncomplicated MI.

In our proposal to the Research Committee we indicated that we would ask the patients who met our criteria for inclusion in the study for their informed consent to randomization on the fifth day after their hospital admission. The Research Committee responded that it had no objection to our performing the clinical trial but that (1) we would have to get permission to include each subject from the patient's attending physician and (2) we were not to mention to the subjects that the length of their stay had been randomized! This ruling—an attempt to avoid increased anxiety for subjects who were felt to be vulnerable to cardiac arrhythmias or other complications associated with stress—indicated the status of thinking on informed consent at the time. We accepted the Research Committee's ruling and did not obtain consent from the subjects. The results of the randomized clinical trial (published in the *New England Journal of Medicine*) indicate that subjects with shorter hospital stays did no worse and probably did better than those who stayed longer. So no harm to subjects was done, other than the lack of respect for their autonomy.

Over the quarter century that I have served as chair of the Montefiore IRB, the pendulum for informed consent has swung dramatically in the opposite direction. Patients are now being asked, for example, to give informed consent for clinical trials for treatment of myocardial infarction within minutes of their arrival in the emergency room, often in a state of acute chest pain and severe anxiety. Protection of subjects' autonomy has taken strong precedence over avoidance of possible harm. In other words, the dictum "first do no harm"[5] has given way to "let the subject decide," even if that process (or the decision made by subjects) may lead to some harm.

It is unlikely that asking for informed consent under these circumstances will itself lead to harm. But there may be other instances in which the principle of autonomy supersedes the principle of nonmaleficence in research involving human subjects. While protection of subjects' autonomy is surely one of the most important criteria in any informed consent process, the other obligations of clinicians may require that IRBs pay closer attention to avoiding harm, even when subjects give consent.

Similar issues of the nature of informed consent, and of risk-benefit analysis, have arisen—with increasing complexity—about research among subjects with HIV infection, among pregnant women, among prisoners, among children, and among subjects without competence or capacity to give informed consent. The roles of IRBs have over the years become more challenging, time-consuming, and often frustrating, and chairing an IRB—either in spite of or because of these new issues—remains an exciting and rewarding experience.

8.B.8 TAKE AWAY MESSAGES

- Chairs should function as enthusiastic leaders; experts on the legal and ethical issues and on federal, state, and local regulations governing research with human subjects and governing IRBs; synthesizers; taskmasters; and diplomats.
- The most important role of IRB chairs is the protection of human subjects, including their right to refuse to participate in research.
- IRB chairs have a duty to ensure that the following elements are included in an informed consent process:
  - Competence,
  - Capacity,
  - Disclosure,

    - Recommendation,
    - Understanding,
    - Decision, and
    - Authorization.
- Chairs must be up-to-date on all regulations and issues surrounding research involving vulnerable subjects.
- IRB chairs provide guidance to inexperienced IRB members and investigators.
- Chairs should:
    - Keep discussion focused,
    - Know when to bring issues to a vote,
    - Table particular discussions until more information becomes available,
    - Consult with IRB resource personnel and craft compromises among group members.

NOTES

1. H. Jonas, *Philosophical Reflections of Experimenting with Human Subjects*, ed. P.A. Freund (New York: George Braziller, 1970).

2. T.L. Beauchamp, J.F. Childress, ed., *Principles of Biomedical Ethics*, 5th ed. (New York: Oxford University Press, 2001).

3. V.W. Sidel, "IRB Oversight of Human Subject Research: Protecting the Subject's Right to Refuse," (presented at a meeting of the Committee on Bioethical Issues of the Association of the Bar of the City of New York, 9 May 2001).

4. Hippocrates, *Decorum* (Cambridge, Mass.: Harvard University Press, 1967), 297.

5. Ibid.

Part C: A Step-by-Step Guide for IRB Members

Lillian Oshva, MD

Part C of chapter 8 is a guide for members of IRBs and will explore the following:

IRBs serve a critical role in protecting human subjects throughout the research process. A thorough IRB review provides protection for potential subjects who are willing to volunteer their bodies to test the efficacy of possible treatments and advance our understanding of diseases.

8.C.1 THE JOB OF THE IRB REVIEWER

The primary reviewer of a study must generally conduct four activities to complete a comprehensive review of a protocol:

1. Gather information:
    - Review study documents, including the study protocol and investigator's brochure,

   - Consult with experts, and
   - Review recent literature.
2. Formulate an overall opinion about the study's potential risk/benefit ratio.
3. Review and make changes to the informed consent document.
4. Consider special populations:
   - Children,
   - Pregnant women,
   - Cognitively impaired persons, and
   - Prisoners.

Lay members are important members of an IRB review and make important contributions in evaluating acceptable risks and benefits for research. Lay members also provide critical guidance by translating scientific concepts into written language in the informed consent document that is clear and informative to the lay public.

8.C.2 PROS AND CONS OF IRB SERVICE

Serving on an IRB can be intellectually challenging and personally rewarding. Physician members of the committee have the opportunity to work closely with professional colleagues from different medical specialties, who, as a result of their diverse training, offer culturally different approaches to problem solving. The opportunity to form personal working relationships and a professional network with such a broad group is often helpful to individual members in their full-time medical practices. Lay members also frequently find these associations rewarding.

Participation on an IRB also exposes members to cutting-edge advances in medicine. Members who review protocols involving experimental drugs learn about new mechanisms of action and possible drug-related toxicities, and become familiar with the "standard of care" for various diseases within disparate medical specialties. Consideration of new devices exposes reviewers to new, creative solutions for fighting disease. Members who review investigator-initiated research often gain expertise in statistical analysis and garner ideas for their own research projects.

On the other hand, the recent national wave of shutdowns by the Office for Human Research Protection (OHRP) and the U.S. Food and Drug Administration (FDA) of research programs at academic medical centers has brought national attention to some of the problems that IRB members can encounter.[1] Board members may face personal liability for board decisions, and workloads on some boards are considerable. IRB service often goes unrewarded in the tenure and promotion arena; a recent article in the *Journal of the American Medical Association* states, "Some IRBs report growing difficulty in attracting dedicated faculty to what is too often a largely thankless job."[2]

8.C.3 NUTS AND BOLTS OF AN IRB REVIEW

Reviewers must complete two sets of work to conduct a thorough IRB review. First, reviewers must develop a point of view on whether the benefits of a research protocol outweigh its potential risks to human subjects, and as a result, whether it deserves approval. Second, reviewers must carefully scrutinize the informed consent document (with special attention focused on the "risks" section) to be certain that the research study and all of the associated understandable dangers have been fully and clearly explained to prospective research subjects.

The actual activities required to complete each of these two tasks often overlap and take place simultaneously. For example, both jobs require that reviewers gain as complete an understanding as possible of a protocol's risks. It is also important, however, to keep these two activities separate in one's mind: it is useless to focus on a protocol's informed consent materials until it is clear that the protocol itself is acceptable when it is evaluated on a risk/benefit basis.

8.C.4 GATHER INFORMATION

There are many possible ways to gather information about a proposed experiment involving human subjects. Industry and cooperative-group sponsored research projects involving an experimental drug will have both an associated investigator's brochure and a study protocol. Device trials or investigator-initiated projects involving drugs that were previously approved by the FDA may only have a study protocol and/or a package insert if the research involves a previously approved drug.

The Investigator's Brochure

The investigator's brochure is the logical place to begin an IRB review. This document is prepared by the industry or cooperative-group sponsor and generally contains technical information about the study's experimental drug or device. Specifically, this document should explain the following:

- The compound's chemical structure.
- Its postulated molecular mechanism of action.
- The various formulations available.
- Results of pharmacokinetic studies in animals and humans, and
- Data from toxicity studies.
- Data from any clinical studies ever conducted that used the drug or the device to treat either the disease in question or other diseases.

Reviewers should try to learn several things from the investigator's brochure. First, they should try to understand the scientific rationale for using this particular compound for this particular disease. Specifically, it is helpful to understand a drug's mechanism of action and the logic for using a drug on the molecular level. Also, it is helpful to understand if there are other drugs on the market or under study that use the same or similar mechanism of action to treat the same disease. If multiple drugs exist within a class of drugs that is under consideration, the relative strengths and weaknesses of the drug under study, when compared to the class, should be understood.

If the disease in question is also treated by other classes of drugs, it is helpful to further understand the advantages and disadvantages of one class of drugs relative to others. While the investigator's brochure may not contain a complete description of other compounds in the same class, or of other classes of drugs used to treat this particular disease, it may begin to outline some relative advantages of its compound over some of the others.

The second set of information that reviewers should look for in the investigator's brochure is data regarding drug safety and side-effects. A key role of reviewers is to understand the known toxicities of an experimental drug as completely as is reasonably possible. This is important both for evaluating a protocol on overall risk/benefit parameters, but also for ensuring that the informed consent document accurately captures known safety issues and possible risks to human research subjects. The investigator's brochure will contain toxicity data from experiments on bacteria, animals, and humans at various drug doses. It is important to understand the results of these previously conducted experiments involving human subjects. These studies may have been conducted to test the experimental drug either for the indication in question or for other unrelated indications.

The third set of data that reviewers can glean from the investigator's brochure relates to the relative efficacy of the compound during any earlier trials conducted for this indication. Any available data about efficacy is likely to be preliminary, but it is generally helpful for reviewers to begin to get a sense of what magnitude of an effect the compound in question could have on disease progression.

Finally, the investigator's brochure may begin to give reviewers a general sense of what unmet needs exist in this particular therapeutic area. To understand unmet needs, reviewers must understand both the severity of the disease in question and the alternatives that are currently available to treat the disease. IRBs may be willing to tolerate a higher-risk profile for a compound or treatment that is aimed at a devastating disease with no known effective therapies, especially in comparison to the risk that would be allowed for an experimental treatment for a benign condition when excellent therapies already exist. Similarly, a "me-too" drug (the fourth or fifth drug in its class for a given indication) may be treated differently than a first-in-class drug that has a novel mechanism of action. Thorough reviewers will understand how the experimental drug in question fits into the universe of clinical need in its therapeutic space and the currently available marketed therapies.

In summary, the investigator's brochure will provide a well-organized reference to much of the information known about the experimental drug in question. Some of this data may not be publicly available. If the trial tests a device, involves no experimental drug, or is investigator-initiated, and there is no investigator's brochure, then reviewers will have to rely on other sources of information and other product information to answer many of these same questions.

The Study Protocol

A second critical document provided to reviewers in all trials is the study protocol. This document outlines the key elements of the proposed study, including the following:

- The study rationale;
- Inclusion and exclusion criteria (to determine eligibility for research subjects entering the study);
- A proposed schedule of study-related activities, including timetables for:
  - Medication doses,
  - Doctors' visits,
  - Tests, and
  - Procedures;
- An explanation of expected study risks; and, finally,
- Proposed primary and secondary therapeutic study endpoints and the statistical methods used to evaluate them.

Thorough reviewers should understand the study schedule so that they can explain to the full IRB what will happen to each subject during each phase of the study. Some IRBs require the principal investigator (PI) to present a study to the committee in lieu of the IRB reviewer. It is helpful for the committee members to understand how the study schedule differs from the routine care that patients with this condition would normally receive. The committee must evaluate the proposed study schedule to ensure, first, that the care provided will be comprehensive enough to approximate the current standard of care, and, second, that any extra tests or procedures required by the study do not pose an unacceptable risk to the research subjects. Further, the committee must ensure that any such risks to the research subjects are clearly outlined in the informed consent document.

Some examples of additional tests or procedures that could pose a risk to research subjects include:

- Invasive procedures such as:
  - Lumbar puncture,
  - Bone marrow biopsy,
  - Endoscopy,
  - Tympanocentesis (puncture of the eardrum),
  - A sham operation, in which a patient is brought to an operating room, a surgeon cuts the patient's skin and pretends to perform an operation, but really does not;
- Imaging techniques that are associated with radiation exposure such as:
  - CT scan,
  - Bone scan,
  - X-ray;
- A "wash-out period," when subjects who already receive therapy for their condition (for example, hypertension, epilepsy, psychiatric condition, et cetera) would be required to go for some time without any medication.

The committee must decide if such risks are acceptable to incur in the context of the research study.

It is important, that reviewers should understand the additional costs that may be associated with any study-related procedure that would not be part of normal patient care, and should have a clear understanding of who will be expected to pay for such extra procedures. Occasionally protocols will be designed with the expectation that research subjects' regular insurance will be billed for particular tests or procedures. In this case, research subjects may be required to spend their own money on additional co-pays or other fees that they would not otherwise incur if they were not study subjects. In the worst-case scenario, subjects may have to pay for the entire cost of a test if their insurance company refuses to pay for a research-related procedure. This can be acceptable to the IRB as long as the informed consent document clearly outlines this risk to subjects. If this provision eliminates the possibility that an investigator can enroll subjects who do not have health insurance, however, an IRB may decide to reject the protocol on the grounds that criteria for the inclusion of human research subjects is not equitable.

Finally, reviewers must evaluate overall inclusion and exclusion criteria for the study. The study should include representatives from as many special groups as possible (women, uninsured persons, children), yet still exclude persons who would be subjected to unacceptably high risks or who would skew the research results.

Overall, the study protocol outlines the actual plan and protocol details that patients and researchers will agree to follow. It should serve as the handbook for the investigator and study coordinator, and is the backbone of IRB reviewers' education about the studies that they will review.

Once reviewers have mastered the material found in these study documents, they should turn to outside sources to confirm the information found in the documents and to fill in gaps in their understanding of the particular disease process and current therapies and treatment processes.

Consult with Experts

Board members will occasionally be asked to review protocols involving diseases or drugs outside of their clinical area of expertise. Medicine has become increasingly sub-specialized, and, in this environment, it is unreasonable to expect a single practitioner to have working knowledge of all medical areas. Reviewers should feel comfortable approaching their professional colleagues for help. Besides tapping friends and acquaintances, reviewers can approach physicians who practice at their own institution— physicians are generally flattered when they are asked to aid in an IRB review by offering their opinions and professional expertise.

Experts can offer insight in various ways. Specifically, board members may use them to gain a more complete understanding of the current standard of care for a disease, including familiarity with procedures routinely used to evaluate patients with a disease, and the therapeutic options that are already available to patients and physicians who manage the disease. Consultants to the full IRB can also contribute to reviews and discussions in a more formal way without voting.

Review Recent Literature

A quick Medline search is convenient and easy to perform and can yield publicly available information about an experimental drug or recent advances and controversies within a therapeutic area. The use of a general internet search engine such as Google can provide a fast overview of currently available treatment options and a comprehensive set of current therapeutic guidelines. Other specialized databases such as the Cochrane Library or ACP Journal Club (at the American College of Physicians web page, *www.acpjc. org*) provide synthesized data about the standard therapies that are currently available. A few institutions are moving to include formal librarian-assisted literature searches as part of the IRB approval process.

8.C.5 FORMULATE AN OVERALL OPINION ON RISK/BENEFIT RATIO

By the time reviewers have gathered information about the disease in question, currently available treatment options, and the proposed experimental drug and research plan, they will probably have a point of view about whether it makes sense to recommend approval of the proposed study by the IRB committee as a whole. To be worthy of committee approval, a project must meet the following requirements.

- The study has an adequate rationale.
- The study has concrete, logical aims and hypotheses.
- It has a methodology that is capable of providing meaningful data with feasible procedures.
- It has a logical timetable or sequence.
- The risks the study will pose to subjects have been minimized.
- The risks are reasonable in relation to any anticipated benefits.
- The selection of subjects will be equitable, with clearly detailed eligibility and exclusionary criteria.
- When appropriate, provisions have been made that are adequate to monitor the data collected to ensure the safety of subjects.
- Adequate provision for the privacy of subjects has been included.[3]

This subject is discussed in greater detail in chapter 2.

If the protocol under consideration is an investigator-initiated project, reviewers may wish to evaluate the statistical validity of any conclusions the protocol is likely to yield. If the proposed study will not have sufficient power to offer a useful result, the potential benefit from the study will be limited. This, of course, will alter the risk/benefit ratio of the research project and may reduce the amount of risk the IRB feels is acceptable for research subjects in a study to assume.

If reviewers have serious concerns about the worthiness of a protocol, it can be helpful for them to gather more information before the meeting so the committee may make a fully informed decision regarding the protocol. Generally, PIs will jump through hoops to return the phone calls of IRB members who call about a submitted protocol, and will usually do so within a few hours. PIs are familiar with the protocol and can clear up procedural questions reviewers may have (for example: confirming that a bone marrow biopsy will only occur if required as a normal part of patient care), and can conceptually agree to appropriate language changes in relevant documents. Such phone calls can often save both PIs and board members weeks of additional wait time and re-reviews while procedural questions are answered, misunderstandings are cleared up, or requests from the committee are considered.

If the protocol under consideration is an industry sponsored or cooperative-group sponsored project, reviewers may wish to consult further with the coordinating physician at the sponsoring organization. This physician will have an even more comprehensive mastery of the study protocol, is eager to help the protocol gain IRB approval, and will be similarly responsive to reviewers' inquiries. If responses do not satisfy reviewers' concerns about a study protocol, IRB members can report with confidence to the larger committee that the protocol should absolutely be rejected.

When reviewers believe the experiment makes sense, it is easy to move forward by recommending approval of the protocol and to begin consideration of the appropriateness of the informed consent form.

8.C.6 REVIEW THE INFORMED CONSENT DOCUMENT

IRB board members may have varying amounts of success in altering study design, but they always have great impact in shaping a protocol's informed consent document. It is the absolute responsibility of an IRB to assure that research subjects have the best chance possible to understand the potential risks and benefits involved in agreeing to participate in a research study.

Although it is often emphasized that informed consent is an entire process, not just a signature on a piece of paper, all would agree that the document itself is an important cornerstone of the process. Subjects will receive a copy of the form to take home after their appointment, and will have the opportunity to review the language that is included in the document with their family and other physicians. It is imperative that the document accurately reflect the study design and be easy to understand. It is generally accepted that the language in the informed consent document should be able to be *understood by a layperson with the reading ability of a sixth grader.*

The "Risks" section of the informed consent document is particularly important in this process. Reviewers should compare the informed consent language with the language and information gathered earlier in the review process when they review study documents, speak with experts, and review the literature.

Many readers have limited attention spans, so the most serious potential risks to a research subject should be explained first in the "Risks" section. Care should be taken to highlight serious risks and avoid burying them between "fainting/bruising from blood draws" and "allergic reactions to EKG stickers." Reviewers should recommend that the informed consent document be formatted in such a way that the individual risks to subjects are clearly separated and highlighted. Overall, the formatting of the document should be used to give the "Risks" section sufficient visual weight.

There are many additional required elements of the informed consent document. The following checklist may be used to evaluate the completeness of an informed consent document.

- A statement that the study involves research is included.
- The reason that subjects have been asked to participate is outlined.
- The expected duration of subjects' participation is included.
- The purpose of the research is stated in lay language.
- The study design is described in lay language.
- Study procedures and treatments are clearly described and match the protocol.
- A description of the drug/device is provided.
- A statement that the drug/device is experimental and has not been approved by the FDA is included (when applicable).
- Any compensation for any injury to subjects that is offered by the sponsor is described.
- Costs to the subjects, if any, for study-related procedures, study medications, et cetera, are outlined.
- The number of subjects in the trial, overall, is disclosed.
- Any possible potential risks and discomforts to subjects is explained in lay language.
- Any potential for direct benefit to subjects and/or benefits to society is outlined.
- Alternatives available to subjects should they choose not to enroll in the study are described.
- A statement that participation is voluntary and that subjects may withdraw at any time without penalty is included.
- A statement regarding confidentiality of research records is included.
- For studies involving drugs, the dosage and route of administration (oral, intravenous, et cetera) is outlined.
- Contact information is provided for subjects who may have questions about the trial.
- Contact information is provided for subjects who have questions regarding their rights as research subjects.
- Contact information is provided for subjects who have questions about research-related injuries.
- Anticipated circumstances under which subjects' participation may be terminated is explained in lay language.
- A statement that significant new findings will be disclosed to research participants is included.
- Any medical consequences of withdrawing from the trial are described.
- The informed consent form does not include any coercive language.
- The informed consent document does not include any exculpatory language (see chapter 3).[4]

8.C.7 CONSIDER SPECIAL POPULATIONS

It is critically important to consider "special populations" in a comprehensive review. These populations have traditionally included groups such as children, psychiatric patients, prisoners, and others who are either unable to make independent decisions or who may be at risk for coercion to participate.

Children

Research involving minors must be categorized into one out of four possible categories by the IRB, and should be evaluated appropriately for corresponding risks/benefits. These categories include:

- Research not involving greater than minimal risk.
- Research involving greater than minimal risk but presenting the prospect of direct benefit to individual subjects.
- Research involving greater than minimal risk with no prospect of direct ben-

efit to individual subjects, but likely to yield generalizable knowledge about the subjects' disease or condition.

- Research that is not otherwise approvable, but which presents an opportunity to understand, prevent, or alleviate a serious problem affecting the health or welfare of children. Research in this last category may be approvable if the IRB consults with a panel of experts who believe that the research presents a reasonable opportunity to a further understanding of disease processes.[5]

Pregnant Women and Fetuses

Pregnant women or fetuses may be involved in research if all of the following conditions are met:

- Similar experiments should first be performed on pregnant animals and non-pregnant women, to obtain data that will help better assess potential risks, when scientifically appropriate.
- To be approvable, a study should either (1) offer potential benefit to the pregnant woman or to the fetus, or to both, or (2) if there is no such potential benefit, the risk to the fetus should be minimal and the research should yield "important biomedical knowledge which cannot be obtained by any other means."[6]
- Risk should be the "least possible for achieving the objectives of the research."[7]
- Informed consent must be obtained from the research subject (the pregnant woman).
- If the research offers potential benefit only to the fetus, the father's informed consent should also be obtained, unless the father is unavailable, incompetent, or temporarily incapacitated. If the pregnancy resulted from either rape or incest, the father's informed consent is similarly not required.
- The research may not offer incentives for terminating a pregnancy.
- "Individuals engaged in the research will have no part in any decisions as to the timing, method, or procedures used to terminate a pregnancy" or in determining the viability of a neonate.[8]

Cognitively Impaired Persons

People in this category have either a psychiatric disorder such as schizophrenia, organic impairment like dementia, or a developmental disorder such as mental retardation that significantly impairs the subject's judgment. If a protocol includes such subjects, the IRB should consider the ability of the potential subjects to give informed consent. The IRB or the protocol may call for the inclusion of an independent clinical monitor to further protect this vulnerable population.

Prisoners

Regulations covering research on subjects in prison are covered in 45 *CFR* 46. There are four categories of allowable research:

1. Studies that involve no more than minimal risk, of the possible causes, effects, and processes of incarceration.
2. Studies that involve no more than minimal risk, of prisons as institutional structures or of prisoners as incarcerated persons. Other studies may be approved if experts in penology, medicine, and ethics approve the study and after written published notice in the *Federal Register.*
3. Research on conditions that are much more prevalent in prisons than elsewhere (such as hepatitis, alcoholism, drug addition, sexual assault).

4. Research on practices that will most likely improve the health or well-being of the subjects. Again, this research may only involve the use of control groups after consultation with appropriate experts in penology, medicine, and ethics, and after written published notice in the *Federal Register.*[9]

In addition, coercion may not be used to enroll prospective prisoner subjects (through better food, living conditions, medical care, et cetera); subject selection must be fair and not controlled by prison authorities; parole boards may not take subjects' participation into consideration; and adequate follow-up care must be provided.

8.C.8 CONTRIBUTIONS FROM NONSCIENTISTS

The lay members of an IRB bring a unique perspective to the review process. They are the only members of the committee who have an understanding of the technical and scientific concepts inherent in the protocol that approximates that of the potential research subjects. As this is the case, lay members have a special responsibility to "translate" technical concepts into regular language that can be clearly understood by the public. Their special responsibility includes simplifying both concepts and individual words. They can also help with formatting documents to insure that information will be easy for potential subjects to understand and access.

In addition, because lay members of an IRB are not familiar or comfortable with many medical procedures, their perspectives on some of the risks and discomforts associated with various medical procedures may differ from that of the physician members of the committee. This perspective is essential to the optimal functioning of the committee.

8.C.9 NEW TECHNOLOGIES

The advent of new technologies has allowed advances in conducting virtual meetings. The use of video-teleconferencing allows board members to meet in two (or more) disparate locations and conduct a meeting in real time. This can cut the inconvenience of commuting for a two-hour meeting, while it preserves the important face-to-face character of regular meetings.

Some IRBs are moving toward paperless processes. Several vendors are developing software that allows boards to provide access to documents in a secure environment through web-based platforms. These new technologies can streamline the board approval process and facilitate the work of IRB members and administrators.

8.C.10 TAKE AWAY MESSAGES

- Pros of serving on an IRB include exposure to cutting-edge medical advances; continuing education in all fields, not just one's own specialty; and forming new relationships that may lead to research collaborations and assistance.
- Cons include the possibility of personal liability for board decisions and additional work,
- Reviewers' jobs include:
  - Gather information
  - Formulate an overall opinion about a study's potential risk/benefit ratio.
  - Review the informed consent document.
  - Consider special populations (children, pregnant women, cognitively impaired persons and prisoners).
- Lay members should evaluate the research from the perspective of the subjects.
- The language in the consent form should be understandable to those with a sixth-grade reading level.

- Make sure all significant side-effects and known potential risks listed in the investigator's brochure are present in the informed consent form.
- Important risks should not be "buried" or minimized in the informed consent form.
- Don't understand something? Ask colleagues, the investigator, or the sponsor for clarification.
- Other good resources are Medline, search engines, the Cochrane Library, or the ACP Journal Club.
- Is this an approvable project? Look for:
    - Adequate rationale.
    - Concrete, logical aims and hypotheses.
    - Methodology capable of producing meaningful data.
    - A logical timetable.
    - Risks to subjects are minimized.
    - Selection of subjects is equitable.
    - Subjects' privacy is protected.

NOTES

1. Johns Hopkins University: S. Levine and R. Weiss, "Hopkins Told to Halt Trials Funded by U.S.; Death of Medical Volunteer Prompted Federal Directive," *Washington Post*, 20 July 2001; J. Bor and T. Pelton, "US Halts Hopkins Research: Most Experiments on Human Subjects Ordered Suspended, Federal Funding Withheld, Oversight Agency Decries Safety Lapses in Volunteer's Death," *Baltimore Sun*, 20 July 2001; "Funds Halted after Asthma Death," *Toronto Star*, 20 July 2001; A. Dembner, "Human Test at Hopkins Halted," *Boston Globe*, 20 July 2001.

Duke University: J.B. Obermayer and S. Cauffman, "US Halts Human Clinical Trials at Duke," *News and Observer*, 12 May 1999; T. Monmaney, "Safety Concerns Suspend Research at Duke Hospital," *Wilmington (N.C.) Morning Star*, 12 May 1999.

The Charles R. Drew University and Science Center and its affiliate, Martin Luther King Jr. Hospital in California: N. Riccardi and T. Monmaney, "King/Drew Medical Research Suspended Health: Voluntary Action Comes After Regulators Find Two Dozen Violations of Rules Designed to Protect Human Subjects and Insurance Credibility at South LA Facility," *Los Angeles Times*, 27 April 2000.

2. J. Moreno et al., "Updating Protections for Human Subjects Involved in Research," *Journal of the American Medical Association* 280, no. 22 (1998): 1956.

3. Biomedical Research Alliance of New York, *Primary Reviewer Checklist* (Great Neck, N.Y.: BRANY, Institute for Research Education, 2002).

4. Biomedical Research Alliance of New York, *Secondary Reviewer Checklist* (Great Neck, N.Y.: BRANY, Institute for Research Education, 2002).

5. 45 *CFR* 46.404-7.

6. *Federal Register*, 66, no. 219 (13 November 2001), Rules and Regulations, pp. 56775-80, via GPO Access, *<wais .access .gpo.gov>< DOCID:fr13no01-9>.*

7. Ibid.

8. Ibid.

9. 45 *CFR* 46.

Part D: The Role of the Institutional Official

Linda Reuter, MS, CIP

The fourth part of this chapter will focus on the role of the institutional official, as follows.

8.D.1 THE OBLIGATIONS AND RESPONSIBILITIES OF INSTITUTIONAL OFFICIALS

The success of any research program relies on institutional support from the highest levels of administration. A quality research program involves a hierarchy of oversight responsibility governed by an institutional official (IO).

The role of the IO is vital in human subjects protections programs. This individual accepts responsibility for the entire oversight program, and must ensure that the institution meets its obligations relating to the conduct of research involving human subjects. For institutions that file a federalwide assurance (FWA),[1] IOs are the individuals who sign the application, and by doing so assume, on behalf of the institution, all of the obligations stated in the FWA document. Therefore, IOs are much more than just "sign offs" for IRB matters.

IOs should be fluent in federal and state regulations, knowledgeable about local policy and procedures for their institution, and cognizant that it is their responsibility with the IRB, sponsors, and investigators, to protect human research participants. IOs must have enough authority to legally represent their institution and allocate the resources needed to ensure adequate support for the institution's human subjects protection program. Generally, an individual at the level of president or chief executive officer of a company, hospital, or health system, or provost, dean, or chancellor of an academic institution, is appropriate for this position. This role may also be delegated to another individual who has the authority to legally represent the institution. IOs should not chair the IRB or be a member of the IRB, nor should they have a clear or perceived conflict of interest. (For example, a director of grants and contracts or anyone whose primary role at the institution is to promote research should not serve as an IO.)

IOs must encourage a high ethical standard of behavior and instill a culture of compliance within their institution. Compliance should be seen not only as doing what regulations say, but doing what is right for subjects. Ethical behavior is the foundation on which a research program should be built, and it will ultimately determine the integrity of the research program. IOs are responsible for ensuring that individuals who conduct research are inspired to do so ethically, and are given adequate opportunity to gain the necessary training and education. IOs typically are responsible for appointing the chair and members of the IRB (or for delegating this responsibility to others), and for allocating appropriate resources and staff to ensure optimal functioning of the IRB.

Identifying an individual to take on this important responsibility is a task that should be taken seriously. If the mission of the institution includes the conduct of research, then high-ranking officials within the institution will understand the significance of having a strong, personal commitment at the highest level of administration. Inadequate institutional support is the number one root cause of compliance problems. Recent headlines related to noncompliance at major research institutions confirm that institutional support and the responsibilities of IOs should not be taken lightly.[2]

IOs are at the top of the reporting structure for IRB matters. Normally, the IRB chair and IRB administrator report to IOs. IOs are the knowledgeable point of contact for the OHRP (for FWA institutions) and are expected to respond to all inquiries from the federal level.

8.D.2 CREATING A CULTURE OF COMPLIANCE

IOs should work closely with IRB chairs, members, and staff to assure development of a comprehensive program to educate all those who are involved in the conduct of research at the institution. IRB staff must be given the resources to provide on-site training programs for researchers, coordinators, IRB members, and anyone else involved in the conduct of research. Additionally, attendance at regional and national meetings related to the protection of human subjects should be encouraged for IRB members, staff, and researchers, so that they will remain current with the rapidly evolving regulatory environment. IOs should encourage participation and, in certain cases, mandate courses and training related to research according to individual roles and responsibilities. IOs should be encouraged to attend these sessions and the IRB meetings as often as possible. IRB members who volunteer their time to serve on the committee will appreciate the presence of IOs. Their presence demonstrates that the institution takes the function of the IRB seriously and that the time spent by its members is recognized. Through an active role in the institution's human subjects protections program, IOs will motivate individuals to become active participants.

IOs can instill a culture of compliance by facilitating presentations at different venues throughout the institution. It is often effective to present IRB and research-related training and education at grand rounds, department and divisional meetings, and even meetings of the board of directors or the medical board. Presentations should be customized for the target audience, ranging from general introductory information (for example: What is an IRB? What does an IRB do? What constitutes research?) to more sophisticated topics for the seasoned researcher (such as: Special considerations for research involving vulnerable populations, Assessing capacity to consent, and so on—this is discussed in more detail in chapter 6.) No employee of any research institution should ever be heard to say, "What is an IRB?" even if they are not directly involved in conducting research.

Providing continuing medical education (CME) credits for completing such training may provide an additional incentive for busy professionals to complete training in IRB and research-related areas, and will encourage compliance with the standard set by IOs (see chapter 6). Once full compliance has been established as an institutional standard, IOs must be diligent in requiring all research staff to meet or exceed this standard. Nothing less can be acceptable.

Such cultures of compliance, with the enthusiastic support of IOs, should enable human subjects protection programs to fulfill their mission.

The goal is a research program that is ethically sound, that is in full compliance with all applicable rules and regulations, and that maximizes the protections for the people who volunteer to participate in research.

8.D.3 TAKE AWAY MESSAGES

- IOs must have enough authority to legally represent their organization and to allocate the resources needed to ensure adequate support for the institution's human subjects protection program.
- Conflicts of interest—perceived as well as actual—must be considered in the selection of an IO. Individuals should not be selected on the basis of how much research they bring to an organization.
- The IRB chair and IRB administrators report to the IO.
- In creating a culture of compliance, education is paramount—use venues such as medical grand rounds and departmental and medical board meetings.

NOTES

1. For more on FWA, see chapter 1. OHRP IRB Registration and Assurance Filing Procedures, *http://www.hhs.gov/ohrp/*, accessed 10 May 2002.

2. Johns Hopkins University: S. Levine and R. Weiss, "Hopkins Told to Halt Trials Funded by U.S.; Death of Medical Volunteer Prompted Federal Directive," *Washington Post*, 20 July 2001; J. Bor and T. Pelton, "US Halts Hopkins Research: Most Experiments on Human Subjects Ordered Suspended, Federal Funding Withheld, Oversight Agency Decries Safety Lapses in Volunteer's Death," *Baltimore Sun*, 20 July 2001; "Funds Halted after Asthma Death," *Toronto Star*, 20 July 2001; A. Dembner, "Human Test at Hopkins Halted," *Boston Globe*, 20 July 2001.

Duke University: J.B. Obermayer and S. Cauffman, "US Halts Human Clinical Trials at Duke," *News and Observer*, 12 May 1999; T. Monmaney, "Safety Concerns Suspend Research at Duke Hospital," *Wilmington (N.C.) Morning Star*, 12 May 1999.

The Charles R. Drew University and Science Center and its affiliate, Martin Luther King Jr. Hospital in California: N. Riccardi and T. Monmaney, "King/Drew Medical Research Suspended Health: Voluntary Action Comes After Regulators Find Two Dozen Violations of Rules Designed to Protect Human Subjects and Insurance Credibility at South LA Facility," *Los Angeles Times*, 27 April 2000.

Part E:
Legal Counsel for Human Subjects Protections Programs

Kendra Dimond, Esq., Mary R. Marta, Esq., and Philip Mitchell, Esq.

The final section of chapter 8 will examine legal considerations, as follows.

8.E.1 HISTORICAL BACKGROUND

Risks and liabilities in clinical research and clinical trials have always been present. There has been a trend recently, however, of increased public interest in the conduct of research involving human subjects. Such interest can be seen in various newspaper articles published across the country regarding prestigious research institutions.[1] The articles are frequently generated as a result of regulatory review of the institution by an oversight agency such as the Department of Health and Human Services (DHHS), Office for Human Research Protections (OHRP) or the Food and Drug Administration (FDA). Publication of newspaper reports and other reports in the literature allow the general public to focus on this particular area of health risk and liability.

For example, in July 2001, the OHRP suspended federally funded research on human subjects at Johns Hopkins University Medical Center following the death of a 24-year-old volunteer during an investigation involving a treatment for asthma. The suspension was lifted three days later. Publications in Baltimore, Washington, D.C., and elsewhere across the country covered the incident and provided the public with information regarding the subject's death.[2]

Johns Hopkins is not the only institution to receive bad publicity for its research. In March 1999, Duke University was found to have issues in its research program after a not-for-cause site visit by the Office of Protection from Research Risks (OPRR).[3] At the time, OPRR halted the enrollment of new subjects in Duke studies for approximately four days and then suspended federally funded research when the school's response to deficiencies cited by the OPRR were deemed to be inadequate.[4] Charles R. Drew University and Science Center and its affiliate, Martin Luther King Jr. Hospital in California (the Center), also had clinical studies stopped after regulators found more than two dozen violations of human research subject protections. The Center placed a self-imposed suspension on its studies, even though such suspension may have threatened the millions of dollars in federal research funds received. According to a newspaper account, federal regulators found that some research projects were not reviewed by the IRB charged with approving them and that such failure to approve was a "major violation."[5]

Public concern over the safety of clinical trials is aroused by harm or death or other unfortunate incidents that occur among the human subjects involved in research studies. A recent review of many clinical trials of new investigational drugs involving children found eight deaths and numerous other adverse events.[6] In one case, an 18-year-old young man who had a mild form of a rare metabolic disorder participated in a gene therapy treatment at the University of Pennsylvania. Within a day of receiving the treatment, the young subject developed serious complications and ultimately died. His death prompted investigations of the trial by the National Institutes of Health (NIH) and the FDA, and the family of the young subject brought suit against the university.[7]

As can be seen by the University of Pennsylvania example, liability associated with clinical research involving human subjects has traditionally focused on the act or omissions of the principal investigator of the research. However, the advent of recent mishaps involving human research subjects has led to greater scrutiny by regulatory authorities and the public of the research activities of those involved at the research institution in the oversight of trials and research. This oversight is typically performed by an IRB.

At the University of Oklahoma Health Sciences Center-Tulsa, the events surrounding the conduct of a melanoma trial raise an uncomfortable awareness of the potential risks of serving on an IRB. The protocol was suspended after an outside audit found major problems, including lack of ongoing oversight by the IRB, and government investigations ensued.[8]

As a result of such scenarios, some participants and their families have become plaintiffs in private litigation.[9] These cases are spearheaded by attorneys who sue the institution, the drug manufacturer, the institutional officials, and, in the Oklahoma case, individual IRB members.[10] These high profile lawsuits have alerted human subjects' and plaintiffs' attorneys to the potential for litigation and have thereby increased the vulnerability of IRBs and their members.

8.E.2 POTENTIAL SOURCES OF LIABILITY

Violation of Law

Failure to comply with appropriate statutes and regulations regarding research is a potential source of liability to the research institution and to its staff, both employees and contractors. The basic DHHS regulation for protection of human research subjects, the "Common Rule," applies to all research involving human subjects that is conducted, supported, or otherwise subjected to the regulation by any federal department or agency that takes appropriate administrative action to make the policy applicable to such research.[11]

The "Common Rule" calls for review of research involving human subjects by an IRB and, by doing so, opens IRBs to potential liability. For example, one of an IRB's major responsibilities is to review the information given to human subjects as part of the informed consent procedure. The "Common Rule" has specific requirements for what an informed consent form must include. However, IRB members, because they see so many informed consent forms, may become acclimated to the language used in informed consent forms and may not always recognize that informed consent language may not be understandable to subjects or subjects' representatives, as required by the "Common Rule." Other flaws in review in informed consent and protocols may also occur.

In addition, IRBs have the responsibility to assure that risks to human subjects are minimized and are reasonable in relationship to the anticipated benefits of a study. This risk/benefit analysis should also include a review of whether such research has been previously reviewed and rejected by other research institutions and IRBs. Such investigations may alert an IRB to a defect in the protocol that it may not have otherwise detected. Although such investigation is not currently mandated under the federal regulations, failure to do so could leave an IRB vulnerable to a claim of common law negligence for failing to exercise reasonable due care in its review of the proposed research study. As of this writing, the FDA is considering enacting such a requirement, and the FDA currently recommends that sponsors provide all pertinent information regarding a proposed research study, including prior IRB denials, to other IRBs for review.[12]

IRBs must also determine whether the selection of subjects is equitable and fair, and must be certain that informed consent, properly documented, will be sought and used. Finally, IRBs must review the research protocol to determine whether adequate provisions to protect human subjects' privacy will be maintained and whether vulnerable subjects, such as children, pregnant women, prisoners, or the mentally ill, will have adequate safeguards in place to protect their rights.

IRBs are authorized to suspend or terminate research that they have previously approved. Suspension or termination may occur when an IRB believes that the research was not conducted in accordance with IRB requirements as part of its ongoing monitoring responsibility. IRBs must report such serious events both internally, to appropriate research institution officials, and externally, to the DHHS through the OHRP (if the institution has an OHRP assurance)[13] and/or to the FDA, if the research concerns a medical device or drug under the FDA's jurisdiction.

IRBs must conduct continuing review of research covered by the "Common Rule" at intervals appropriate to the degree of risk of the research. This requires that IRBs continually monitor the risks that human subjects may face and take appropriate action when such risks may be elevated during the course of the research, although not foreseen at the time of approval.

Deficiencies in compliance with law and regulation by an IRB can trigger administrative actions against an institution resulting in criminal or civil sanctions by the FDA or an investigation by the DHHS Office of the Inspector General (OIG) and the U.S. Department of Justice. When there is apparent noncompliance that creates a significant threat to the rights and welfare of human subjects, the FDA may notify relevant state and federal regulatory agencies and other parties with a direct interest in the agencies' actions of the deficiencies in the operations of the IRB.[14] Institutions that receive NIH funding must certify in applications and progress reports that they are complying with human subjects regulations and that all information that they have provided to the government is true. In cases of noncompliance or inaccurate reporting, the government could allege that false statements or claims to the government have been made, and may bring civil or criminal charges.[15]

Although the above has primarily been a discussion of the federal law concerning potential violations of the law by IRBs or research institutions, there are state and local laws that may affect how research may be performed within a jurisdiction. An institution or independent IRB should make itself aware of these laws before it commences clinical research activities.

Violation of Contract

The prevailing priority among study sponsors, principal investigators, study sites, and IRBs, from a risk-management perspective, is compliance with applicable federal regulations regarding the conduct of a clinical research study. However, in addition to regulatory compliance, IRBs must be mindful to include contractual liability in their risk analysis. Contractual liability may arise in one of two important contexts.

First, contractual relationships between a non-institutionally based IRB (subsequently referred to as an "independent IRB") and the study site (or between research institutions regarding use of an internal IRB for oversight of trials conducted under a cooperative research agreement) may create additional risks for the contracting parties if they are not closely monitored. In circumstances where an IRB adopts more stringent practice standards than required under applicable law or community standards—whether voluntarily or through the negotiation process with the study site—the IRB will be held to the higher standards in the face of injury to study participants arising from the study.

For example, an IRB operating under FDA regulations is required to conduct continuing review of approved studies not less than annually.[16] If, however, an IRB assumes the responsibility of monthly reviews under its agreement with a study site, the IRB could be contractually liable if it conducts ongoing reviews less frequently, when its failure to conduct ongoing reviews as scheduled causes it to fail to detect a problem in the study that results in injury to a subject. The IRB's liability under these circumstances could be further exacerbated if its promise to utilize the higher standards was a significant factor in the study site's selection of that IRB over other IRBs.

These contractual liabilities may arise whether or not an IRB's arrangement with the study site is documented in writing. Although federal regulations do not require written agreements between an independent IRB and a study site,[17] it is essential, from a risk-management standpoint, that each IRB routinely require a signed agreement before undertaking the review of a study that is not based at its institution. These contracting formalities may easily be overlooked, particularly by internal IRBs that only sporadically undertake oversight of clinical research outside of their institution.

Such contracts permit the parties to expressly set forth their respective responsibilities and establish a clear process for ongoing communication during the conduct of a study. In addition, they allow the parties to document compliance with the confidentiality requirements established under applicable law, including, but not limited to, the federal regulations recently adopted under the Health Insurance Portability and Accountability Act (HIPAA).[18] Furthermore, in such settings, communication between an IRB's contract negotiator and its IRB administrator is of critical importance. Lack of such coordination would leave the IRB in the unenviable position of not being able to fulfill its contractual obligations without significant additional costs or operational inconvenience.

Second, institutions with internal IRBs could face similar issues with their research administrators, whether their responsibilities are documented in a formal employment or independent contract agreement or written job description, if the document does not reflect actual practice. Contracting parties often tend not to review their written obligations once the agreement is negotiated and signed. However, if the parties' collective practice during the term of the arrangement varies significantly from the terms of the contract or job description, and adherence to the written standards may have prevented or diminished a subject's injury, each party may ultimately be liable for failing to abide by its contractual obligations.

While study subjects are not parties to the IRB agreements described above (either under a sponsored research agreement or an agreement between a research institution and its IRB administrator), these documents may be critical in assessing liability of the parties for a subject's injury during a trial. These agreements will serve as the standard to judge whether each party's acts (and omissions) were reasonable under a traditional negligence theory. In addition, it is not inconceivable that an injured study subject might attempt to recover damages for a party's breach of the IRB agreement as a third-party beneficiary to the contract.

For a subject to succeed as a third-party beneficiary under a breach of contract theory, the contracting parties must have intended to directly benefit the third party. Since the central function of any IRB's trial oversight is to assure that the rights, safety, and welfare of the study subjects are protected, it may be possible for an injured subject to maintain a claim on these grounds. Because of the potential risk of contractual liability, an independent IRB's precise role and function in each research study should be well documented, so that the IRB is in a position to judge the risk it may be undertaking and to adequately protect itself, to the extent possible, through insurance and indemnification, as discussed below in greater detail.

Violation of IRB Policy

Recruitment for the difficult and time-consuming task of being an IRB member may become even more difficult if potential members fear liability from these types of legal actions. This may result in a hesitancy to approve controversial and cutting-edge medical research. The allegations made in recent civil actions go beyond the requirements of federal or state law and attack the institutional policies under which research is conducted.

For example, the failure to disclose financial relationships with sponsors has been alleged as a negligent abrogation of informed consent, under the theory that it constituted a failure to warn human subjects of a bias held by the researchers that could affect objectivity in the conduct of research. Such an allegation was made in the previously mentioned gene therapy case, which was quickly settled out of court by the University of Pennsylvania.[19] Financial relationships between the researchers, the institution, and a product manufacturer, undisclosed to subjects, form the basis for allegations in currently ongoing litigation brought by research subjects and families against the Fred Hutchinson Cancer Research Center in Seattle, Washington.[20]

IRBs, when they approve protocols and consent forms, become a potential defendant for this allegation. A focus on recruitment of investigators would find ample evidence of financial incentives.[21] Should IRBs insist that human subjects be told of any and all relationships between investigators and sponsors? Research institutions themselves could have a financial relationship with sponsors. Should subjects be made aware of that also? IRBs may decide that, as a matter of policy, this must occur. If so, they must also decide if they will draw limits under which the information is not reportable to subjects. For federally funded research, the NIH demands that a conflict of interest committee review reportable relationships and decide what management of a potential conflict of interest need occur.[22] The FDA requires that, for research it regulates, the sponsor must report financial relationships with investigators.[23] However, under neither federal reporting requirement is there a duty to communicate this information to subjects.

Of course, not all conflict of interest is financial. There is an inherent risk that the investigative goal of the researcher conflicts with the therapeutic expectations of the subjects, and that this might manifest itself in the informed consent process. IRBs must be sensitive to this issue and consider policies to avoid undue pressure by the researcher.

Recent federal legislative activity, prompted by the events at the University of Pennsylvania, Johns Hopkins, and the University of Oklahoma, as discussed earlier, may alter this scenario. A House Bill introduced on 9 May 2002 (H.R. 4697) would require investigators to disclose their conflict of interest to IRBs and to potential subjects. This same bill would also apply the "Common Rule" to all human research subjects, independent of setting and funding source, and it would authorize the DHHS to impose sanctions, including withholding federal funding from IRBs.

State laws may impose duties involving conflict of interest and human subject protections generally and must be reviewed by IRBs to ensure that their policies are compliant. For example, a California court held that the failure to disclose a financial interest held by a physician in the body fluids of a patient could give rise to a cause of action for performing medical procedures without informed consent, or for a breach of fiduciary duty.[24] The physician was conducting research on cells obtained from the patient. Under the California law, a physician who plans to conduct a medical experiment on a patient must inform the patient of the sponsor or funding source for the experiment.[25]

The pending federal legislation does not pre-empt state laws, so multi-state clinical trials would still be governed by varying standards. This highlights the IRB policy issue, that is, whether to adopt a standard that is stricter than federal law, or even state law, using a "best practices" approach and so hope to avoid litigation, while providing additional protections for human subjects. IRBs must consider the cost of such enhanced policies and procedures and the burden of initiating them, compared with the benefits and protections they would provide to the subjects, the researchers, and the institution. Sometimes institutions believe this is best accomplished by reducing the number of trials that an IRB reviews and turning over review of multi-center studies, in particular, to an independent for-profit IRB. Other institutions, while enhancing their policies and procedures, have also increased the number of their internal IRBs.

On 15 April 2002, in apparent recognition of efforts made by research institutions under its federalwide assurance process (FWA) to identify best practices, the OHRP published a description of its quality improvement program for human subject research.[26] On 4 April 2002, the OHRP published a set of guidelines for IRB procedures.[27] The guidelines describe more fully the information that IRBs should review and document, review common findings of OHRP noncompliance, give guidance on expedited review, and encourage compliance with other federal policies such as the inclusion of women and minorities in research.

On the topic of conflict of interest, the guidance addresses conflicts of interest and recusal regarding members of IRBs, but does not discuss whether or not an IRB should insist that researchers disclose real or potential conflicts to subjects. Once again, IRBs must make this policy decision.

An IRB may find itself accused of approving a protocol that it should not have approved, based on a court's review of the protocol during litigation. The IRB may think it has followed the federal and state guidelines, and thus believe that it is protected; however, one recent decision is illustrative of why that is not always so. In late 2001 the Maryland Court of Appeals examined a case in which families with young children became subjects in nontherapeutic research involving lead abatement procedures for paint in housing.[28] After some children began to experience difficulties, two suits were brought against the institution conducting the research. The trial courts dismissed the cases, finding no legal duty to warn the children or parents of the risk.

In reinstating the two suits, the Maryland Court of Appeals took a dim view of the nontherapeutic study, particularly since children were involved and their parents were giving consent. The court found that informed consent agreements can constitute contracts, that a duty of care can arise out of the research/subject relationship, and that breach of that duty can constitute negligence. The court also held that a parent cannot consent to a child's participation in a nontherapeutic study in which there was more than the minimal risk of everyday life.

The court remanded the case for further factual development of the issues relating to potential liability or damages. In May 2002, the Maryland legislature passed a law requiring all persons conducting research involving human subjects to comply with federal regulations on the protection of human subjects and that IRB minutes must be made available for inspection upon request. (Confidential or privileged information may be removed.)[29]

The foregoing scenario should not be viewed in isolation. Given that IRBs often operate independently without direct oversight from a research institution, it is not inconceivable that an IRB could approve a research study beyond the scope of its authority. For example, an IRB could approve a study involving children, even though the institution does not have a strong pediatrics program. Therefore IRBs, particularly internal IRBs, must be aware of their institutions' general policies and restrictions on the types of research that are permitted to be carried out there. Failure to understand these restrictions could result in potential liability both for the research institution and the IRB.

8.E.3 LIABILITY ISSUES

Who Is Liable?

While they are arguably one of the most important players in the conduct of clinical trials, IRBs are perhaps the least visible to study subjects. Study subjects will, in most instances, have direct contact with the principal investigator and study site, will know the sponsor, and may potentially have contact with the contract research organization (CRO) or site management organization (SMO), if they are utilized by the sponsor. Because an IRB's primary function is to safeguard the interests of the study subjects involved in a study at a particular site, IRBs (whether independent or internal) and their members face a potential risk of liability for their role in the study if complications arise. Despite IRBs' vital role in monitoring a clinical research study, federal regulations do not immunize IRBs or individual IRB committee members from liability for their actions that are taken as part of their oversight function. In fact, the FDA has publicly acknowledged that it has no authority to limit the potential liability of IRBs or their members.[30] Since immunity from liability is not provided under law, IRBs and their members need to be fully cognizant of the circumstances under which they could be held liable for their actions in participating in clinical trial review oversight.

An independent IRB or the research institution that supports an internal IRB may be vicariously liable for the acts of its individual committee members who oversee a study. Under the common law theory of respondent superior, a "master" is responsible for the acts of its "servant." While there is no definitive or universally accepted test to determine whether a master-servant relationship exists, courts generally employ a multifactor test, with the determining factor being the master's right to control the ongoing details of the servant's work. For example, an employer-employee relationship clearly falls within this category. Similarly, in most instances, individual IRB members, based on their activities as members of a committee, would likely be determined to be under the control of the entity, even when the IRB members are not strictly "employees" of the IRB (or its institution). In fact, payment for services is not required for a finding that a master-servant relationship exists. Therefore, under the appropriate circumstances, an entity can be held liable for the acts (or omissions) of its volunteers.

Where the master-servant relationship exists, the master may be liable for both the negligent and intentional acts of its servants. However, where the servant's actions are motivated by personal interests unrelated to the business purpose or mission of the master, the master may escape liability for the servant's negligence and/or intentional acts. For example, it is unlikely that an independent IRB or research institution would be held responsible for an IRB member's negligent activity in approving a study, when the IRB member knowingly failed to disclose to the independent IRB (or institution) that he or she had a financial interest in the study sponsor. Subject to that exception, an IRB will likely be liable for its committee members' negligent and intentional acts that have been undertaken in furtherance of the IRB's mission.

The foregoing scenario should not be confused, however, with a study site's liability for the negligent acts of an independent IRB. When an IRB is engaged as an independent contractor by a study site, the study site generally will not be liable for the acts or omissions of the IRB, because the study site does not have the right to control the manner in which the IRB performs its oversight responsibilities. However, if a court determined that the IRB's work is inherently risky or dangerous, or that the study site had a nondelegable duty to protect the safety of its subjects, the study site could be held vicariously liable for the IRB's acts, even though an independent contractor relationship exists. In addition, the institution or practice could conceivably be held partially liable for the acts of the independent IRB if the study site did not use due care and reasonable judgment in selecting the particular IRB to oversee the conduct of the study.

For institutions that use internal IRBs that also rely on independent IRBs, the issue of liability may be further clouded under the institution's FWA with OHRP (when applicable). The OHRP requirement to file an FWA includes both "awardee" and collaborating "performance site" institutions. The awardee institution has ultimate responsibility for protecting human subjects under a DHHS award and must ensure that all collaborating institutions also hold an OHRP approved assurance.[31] Under an FWA, the study site remains responsible for ensuring compliance with the terms of its FWA, as well as the determinations of the reviewing IRB.

At this point in time, an individual IRB member's personal liability is unclear. To date, there is no known reported holding in which an IRB member has been held personally liable for his or her actions involving conduct of a clinical research study. The authors were eagerly anticipating the outcome of the University of Oklahoma litigation to see if the court would find IRB members personally liable in that case.[32] However, this suit was settled regarding the institution and IRB members without public comment by the litigants. The authors cannot predict what will happen in the future regarding individual IRB member liability. If an IRB member undertakes his or her responsibilities in good faith, however, it appears unlikely at present that she or he will be held personally liable for participating in IRB functions, whether as a volunteer member or paid employee or consultant.

Insurance Coverage

Insurance coverage may be obtained in many ways. Examples include coverage through a commercial insurer, a self-insurance trust, or a captive insurance company owned by a research institution. Coverage under each type of insurance varies, particularly insurance policies purchased from commercial insurers. Because of this variability in insurance coverage, it is important for research institutions and those involved in research, including IRB members, to review their coverage with an institutional representative, such as the chief financial officer (CFO), risk manager, or director of research, and a representative of the insurance company, trust, or captive. Professional liability (that is, malpractice) coverage, directors and officers policies, general liability coverage, umbrella insurance policies, and other forms of coverage should be reviewed to determine the scope of research activities covered and the personnel that each policy covers and/or excludes.

In terms of personnel, IRB members may include research institution employees, independent contractors, and community volunteers. Merely having such policies is not enough; risk managers must read the fine print of the policies to understand who is covered and under what circumstances. Insurance policy boilerplate language may be insufficient to meet a research institution's or IRB's particular needs. Once the institution and those involved in research determine whether or not coverage is provided, appropriate action can be taken. If coverage is not provided, the research institution and/or the IRB members and others involved in research should consider purchasing insurance that will cover the research risks involved.

An institution's malpractice policy may cover some allegations of harm under the theory that it occurred in relation to the care of patients, but malpractice policies generally do not cover officers and directors, IRB members, nonemployed physicians, or other non-healthcare providers. Other policies that need to be reviewed for possible coverage in the event of clinical trial litigation include the general liability policy for bodily injuries, and directors' and officers' policies for breach of fiduciary duty. The institution's existing policies need to be examined for error and omissions coverage and products liability coverage. Indemnification costs may be covered by insurance also.

There is an underlying distinction between the goals of research and the risk-benefit analysis normally performed in standard patient care. Not surprisingly, sponsors and institutions are now seeking separate clinical trial coverage. Some underwriters are asking investigators and IRB members for proof of formal training or accreditation in doing clinical trials. Institutions are also requesting indemnification for their IRB members from trial sponsors. Clinical trial insurance can be a part of a general liability policy or a separate policy. In particular, an institution would want non-physician investigators, non-employees, and IRBs covered by such a policy, as well as any indemnification to the sponsors.[33]

The Risk Retention Act of 1986 made it possible for larger entities to self-insure.[34] Many institutions did so and used established insurance companies only for insurance in excess of their limit. Institutional administrators must examine whether the IRB can be named as an additional insured under such policies, keeping in mind the risks versus the cost of the insurance.

Indemnification

In the wake of the previously discussed, well-published serious adverse events in several trials around the country, IRB members have been increasingly sensitive to the potential liability exposure they may face that arises from participation in IRB functions. Despite these recent developments, to this point no IRB member has ever been subject to personal liability for serving in such capacity. As long as IRB members serve in good faith and without deliberate dishonesty, personal liability for IRB participation remains unlikely. That being said, however, IRBs as well as their individual members should be familiar with the circumstances under which they may be indemnified (that is, reimbursed) for costs that they may incur from claims arising from their participation in research activities.

In light of the current law, the costs for IRB members would most likely involve the cost of engaging an attorney to extricate the IRB member from a lawsuit rather than payment of damages to a successful plaintiff. The right to indemnification may arise from contract or by law, and the source of the indemnification obligation may vary from the independent IRB or a research institution (for an internal IRB) to a third party, such as the CRO, SMO, or sponsor, depending on the circumstances of the particular construct of the clinical research study.

Generally speaking, officers and directors of an entity, acting in their official capacities, may be indemnified by the entity for which they provide their services. Such indemnification rights are often contained in an entity's charter, bylaws, or both. These provisions may provide detailed procedures for the circumstances under which the entity will and will not provide indemnification to its officers and directors or may simply recite that indemnification will be provided to the extent permitted by applicable law.

In New York, for example, both the business corporation law and the not-for-profit corporation law permit indemnification by an organization for the costs and expenses incurred by its officers and directors in defending third-party actions, except to the extent the act giving rise to the claim or injury resulted from an individual's bad faith, deliberate dishonesty, or when he or she received financial gain or other advantage to which he or she was not entitled.[35] These types of statutory indemnification provisions often require corporate indemnification when the corporate officer or director is successful in defending the third-party claim, even when not specifically permitted by the entity's organizational documents. Thus, corporate officers and directors are generally well protected for acts they perform in their official capacities.

While an entity's officers and directors are generally well protected under these indemnification provisions and statutes, other corporate representatives, such as volunteers or non-director members, may not enjoy such statutory indemnification protection.[36] Therefore, independent IRBs and institutions should review their corporate organizational documents and state law to confirm that all IRB members are entitled to the same level of indemnification. To the extent the IRB members' indemnification rights are not consistent, appropriate changes should be implemented.

This may be accomplished in several ways, whether through individual agreements, organization documents, and/or duly adopted policy. It is not unusual, for example, to see identical indemnification provisions in an institution's corporate bylaws (with respect to its officers and directors) and its medical staff bylaws (with respect to medical staff members for action taken as a member of a medical staff or institution-wide committee). With respect to individuals who may not be specifically covered by the entity's organizational documents, such as volunteers and consultants, the independent IRB and institution would be wise to adopt a specific policy to address the indemnification of such IRB members. Courts will typically uphold such indemnification obligations undertaken by contract or policy, to the extent otherwise permitted under law. However, courts may not enforce indemnification agreements where payment is deemed to violate public policy.

For example, many states will not honor indemnification obligations that include payment for punitive damages, because such awards are generally based on personal misconduct or bad faith. Furthermore, potential IRB members should be fully apprised of the indemnification policy of the independent IRB or institution (if any) as part of the new member orientation, so that such individuals are fully informed of the potential exposure they may face prior to committing to participation in IRB activities.[37]

An IRB's potential exposure for risks attendant with a clinical research study may be limited by an indemnification provision in the clinical study agreement (or the written agreement between the external IRB and the study site). In the event that the study is overseen by an internal IRB, the general indemnity provision contained in the study agreement should be broadly drafted to cover the ongoing activities of the internal IRB. This issue can be easily overlooked since the parties to the clinical study agreement—typically the institution and principal investigator and the sponsor and CRO—often are not focused on the internal IRB's ongoing role in the study.

Contractual indemnification provisions tend to be heavily negotiated during the contracting phase, but serve the collective interest of the parties such that each party is responsible to the other party for its own actions (or omissions).[38] Absent such agreement, the wronged party may sue the other party for costs arising from the other party's action, and several states have adopted the Uniform Contribution Among Tortfeasors Act to establish a clear standard for apportioning liability among the parties, based on their relative culpability.

Other Liability Protection Issues

The breakdown of human subjects protections during a clinical trial could lead to substantial liability in damages to subjects and their families, as well as to governmental investigations and penalties. In addition, a failure to have proper protocols in place could lead to sponsors' liability, either directly or under an indemnification provision.

Most importantly, an IRB must adhere strictly to its written policies and procedures and revisit these documents frequently to ensure that (1) human subjects protections are intact and adequate, (2) the IRB understands the scope of its authority, and (3) it effectively communicates these policies and rules to its members to ensure that they are implemented properly. At a time when advertising and recruitment for trial participation is ever increasing, diligence on the part of IRBs is imperative. The possibility of public or private influx of funding that accompanies clinical research may encourage researchers and institutions to use highly aggressive methods to advertise or recruit. IRBs must carefully review these methods to ensure that federal guidelines are followed and to protect against any future allegations of misrepresentation or fraud.[39]

8.E.4 OTHER ISSUES

The independence of IRBs has traditionally been emphasized, since they must oversee research without bias or duress from any party. However, liability accusations make no such distinction, and an IRB and its members may find themselves as codefendants with the researcher, the bioethicist, and the institution or other research sites. Often privately sponsored trials are conducted outside institutional settings, and the protocols are reviewed by independent IRBs.[40]

If an IRB is a separate, nonprofit entity, it must have procedures to monitor itself for compliance with federal and state law and policy. However, when an IRB is composed primarily of employees of an institution, the institution must ensure that it is protecting itself by monitoring its IRB's compliance. Some institutions do this by having in-house counsel or another management-level person on the IRB or attending meetings. When this occurs, caution must be taken not to abrogate the IRB's function. Often this is accomplished by assuring that such institutional officials are nonvoting members and are recused when appropriate.

A CRO can be pulled into the liability net also. CROs may be involved in recruiting subjects, designing trials, or actual trial procedures. They are traditionally paid by pharmaceutical companies in privately sponsored trials, and must guard against the inherent bias that arises from that relationship. IRBs must interact with CROs to ensure that human subjects are protected, and that the rights and obligations of each party in the research study—that is, of the IRB, the sponsor, the practice site, and the CRO—are expressly stated and understood.

8.E.5 TAKE AWAY MESSAGES

- High-profile lawsuits have alerted human subjects' and plaintiffs' attorneys to the potential for litigation and have thereby increased the vulnerability of IRBs and their members.
- To date, there is no known reported holding in which an IRB member has been held personally liable for his or her actions involving conduct of a clinical research study. However, the authors cannot opine on what may happen in the future regarding the liability of individual IRB members.
- IRBs must be cognizant of their organization's general policies on the types of permitted research.
- IRBs should be sure that their standard operating procedures (SOPs) are current and that all members and staff adhere to those policies.
- The use of an external IRB may not protect a study site from potential liability.
- IRBs should be mindful to include contractual liability in their risk analysis.
- IRBs should ensure that sponsors indemnify their members when contracts are negotiated.
- IRBs should ensure adequate liability coverage for their members.
- IRB members should be appraised of their responsibilities as IRB members and of their organization's indemnification policies.

NOTES

1. Johns Hopkins University: S. Levine and R. Weiss, "Hopkins Told to Halt Trials Funded by U.S.; Death of Medical Volunteer Prompted Federal Directive," *Washington Post*, 20 July 2001; J. Bor and T. Pelton, "US Halts Hopkins Research: Most Experiments on Human Subjects Ordered Suspended, Federal Funding Withheld, Oversight Agency Decries Safety Lapses in Volunteer's Death," *Baltimore Sun*, 20 July 2001; "Funds Halted after Asthma Death," *Toronto Star*, 20 July 2001; A. Dembner, "Human Test at Hopkins Halted," *Boston Globe*, 20 July 2001.

Duke University: J.B. Obermayer and S. Cauffman, "US Halts Human Clinical Trials at Duke," *News and Observer*, 12 May 1999; T. Monmaney, "Safety Concerns Suspend Research at Duke Hospital," *Wilmington (N.C.) Morning Star*, 12 May 1999.

The Charles R. Drew University and Science Center and its affiliate, Martin Luther King Jr. Hospital in California: N. Riccardi and T. Monmaney, "King/Drew Medical Research Suspended Health: Voluntary Action Comes After Regulators Find Two Dozen Violations of Rules Designed to Protect Human Subjects and Insurance Credibility at South LA Facility," *Los Angeles Times*, 27 April 2000.

2. See note 1 above.

3. The DHHS moved OPRR, formerly under the NIH, to the supervision of the DHHS itself. It is now the Office for Human Research Protections (OHRP).

4. See note 1 above.

5. Ibid.

6. A. Dembner, "Dangerous Dosage," *Boston Globe*, 18 February 2001.

7. *Gelsinger v. University of Pennsylvania*, Philadelphia County Court of Common Pleas, Term 2000 (Complaint filed 19 September 2000; settled 4 November 2000).

8. J. Washburn, "Informed consent, *Robertson v. The University of Oklahoma Health Services Center-Tulsa*," *Washington Post Magazine*, 30 December 2001, p. 10.

9. Ibid.

10. *Robertson et al. v. McGee et al.*, U.S.D.C., N.D. Oklahoma No. 01CV00GOH (M).

11. 45 *CFR* Part 46.

12. See 21 *CFR* 56.109 (e) and *FDA IRB Information Sheet-Guidance for Institutional Review Boards and Clinical Investigators: Frequently Asked Questions* (1998 update). This FDA IRB Information Sheet can be found at *www.fda.gov/oc/ohrt/frbs/freqs.html.*

13. Every institution engaged in research involving human subjects that is supported or conducted by the DHHS must have an assurance of compliance approved by OHRP. See 45 *CFR* § 46.103.

14. 21 *CFR* § 56.120.

15. See: *United States ex rel Chandler v. The Hecktoen Institute for Medical Research*, 35 F.Supp. 2d 1078 (1999), U.S.C.A., 7th Circuit, Nos. 00-4110 and 01-1810, 22 January 2002 (institute accused of misrepresenting compliance with human subjects regulations in grant progress report). See also *United States v. Stephen Breuning*, C. No. K-88-0135 (D.MD) 1988 (researcher at the University of Pittsburgh charged with submitting false information in National Institute of Mental Health (NIMH) grant renewal pleaded guilty to making two false statements).

16. See 21 *CFR* § 56.108 (f).

17. See *FDA IRB Information Sheet-Guidance for Institutional Review Boards and Clinical Investigators: Non-Local IRB Review* (1998 update). This FDA IRB Information Sheet can be accessed online at *www.fda.gov/oc/ohrt/irbs/nonlocal review.html.*

18. For the FDA confidentiality requirements, see 21 *CFR* § 56.111(a)(7) and 21 *CFR* § 50.25(b)(5). Under the HIPPA regulations, covered healthcare providers are required to maintain agreements with their business associates regarding the confidentiality of individually-identifiable health information regarding patients to which the business associates may have access. See generally, 45 *CFR* § 164.502(e). Note: research study participants may also be subjected to additional confidentiality requirements under the state law.

19. See note 7 above.

20. *Wright v. The Fred Hutchinson Cancer Research Center et al.*, U.S.D.C., W.D. Washington, No. C01-5217 (2001).

21. See DHHS, OIG, *Recruiting Human Subjects: Pressures in Industry-Sponsored Clinical Research* (Washington, D.C.: DHHS, June 2000, Pub. No. OE-01-97-000193).

22. The specific NIH reportable relationships are set forth in 42 *CFR* Part 50, Subpart F.

23. The specific FDA reportable financial relationships are explained in 21 *CFR* Part 54.

24. *Moore v. Regents of the University of California*, 271 Cal. Rptr. 146, 793 P. 2d 479 (1990).

25. Health & Safety Code *§ 24173*

Health & Safety, subd. (c) (9).

26. *http://ohrp.osophs.dhhs.gov/humansubjects/qup/qipdesc.pdf.*

27. *http://ohrp.osophs.dhhs.gov/compovr.htm.*

28. *Grimes v. Kennedy Krieger Institute, Inc.*, 782A 2d 807 (Md. 2001).

29. House Bill 917, 16 May 2002.

30. *See FDA IRB Information Sheet-Guidance for Institutional Review Boards and Clinical Investigators: Frequently Asked Questions* (1998 update). This FDA IRB Information Sheet can be accessed online at *www.fda.gov/oc/ohrt/irbs/faqs.html.*

31. See *IRB Registration and Assurance Filing Procedures, http://ohr.osophs.dhhs.gov/humansubjects/assurance/refinfo.htm.*

32. For further discussion of the University of Oklahoma litigation, see "8.E.1 Historical Background," in this chapter.

33. See "8.E.3: Indemnification" in this chapter.

34. Public Law 99-563. The Risk Retention Act of 1986 is codified at 15 *U.S.C.* 3901 et seq.

35. See N.Y. Business Corporation Law § § 721-724 and N.Y. Not-for-Profit Corporation Law § § 721-724.

36. Note: the corporation law of some states, such as Pennsylvania, expressly provide certain indemnification rights for all corporate representatives, not only officers and directors. See 15 P.S. § § 1741, 1743.

37. Note: the IRB's indemnification obligations (whether by charter or contract) may be funded by some form of insurance. As part of the IRB's review of its indemnification policies, it would be advisable to also review its insurance coverage to ensure that its indemnification obligations (i.e., contractual liabilities) are covered.

38. A research institution or site has the right of indemnification under contract and should require a certificate of insurance from the sponsor or CRO, if applicable, to ensure that the sponsor can meet its contractual liabilities.

39. See note 21 above.

40. DHHS, OIG, *Institutional Review Boards: The Emergence of Independent Boards* (Washington, D.C.: DHHS, June 1998, Pub. OEI-01-97-00192).

Appendix A
The Nuremberg Code

Excerpted from "Permissable Medical Experiments," Trials of War Criminals before the Nuernberg Military Tribunals under Control Council Law No. 10: Nuernberg, October 1946 -1949, *vol. 2 (Washington, D.C.: U.S. Government Printing Office, n.d.), 181-2.*

1. The voluntary consent of the human subject is absolutely essential. This means that the person involved should have legal capacity to give consent; should be so situated as to be able to exercise free power of choice without the intervention of any element of force, fraud, deceit, duress, overreaching, or other ulterior form of constraint or coercion; and should have sufficient knowledge and comprehension of the elements of the subject matter involved as to enable him to make an understanding and enlightened decision. This latter element requires that before the acceptance of an affirmative decision by the experimental subject there should be made known to him the nature, duration, and purpose of the experiment; the method and means by which it is to be conducted; all inconveniences and hazards reasonably to be expected; and their effects upon his health or person which may possibly come from his participation in the experiment.

The duty and responsibility for ascertaining the quality of the consent rests upon each individual who initiates, directs, or engages in the experiment. It is a personal duty and responsibility which may not be delegated to another with impunity.

2. The experiment should be such as to yield fruitful results for the good of society, unprocurable by other methods or means of study, and not random and unnecessary in nature.

3. The experiment should be so designed and based on the results of animal experimentation and a knowledge of the natural history of the disease or other problem under study that the anticipated results will justify the performance of the experiment.

4. The experiment should be so conducted as to avoid all unnecessary physical and mental suffering and injury.

5. No experiment should be conducted where there is an *a priori* reason to believe that death or disabling injury will occur, except perhaps, in those experiments where the experimental physicians also serve as subjects.

6. The degree of risk to be taken should never exceed that determined by the humanitarian importance of the problem to be solved by the experiment.

7. Proper preparations should be made and adequate facilities provided to protect the experimental subject against even remote possibilities of injury, disability or death.

8. The experiment should be conducted only by scientifically qualified persons. The highest degree of skill and care should be required through all stages of the experiment of those who conduct or engage in the experiment.

9. During the course of the experiment the human subject should be at liberty to bring the experiment to an end if he has reached the physical or mental state where continuation of the experiment seems to him to be impossible.

10. During the course of the experiment the scientist in charge must be prepared to terminate the experiment at any stage, if he has probable cause to believe, in the exercise of the good faith, superior skill, and careful judgment required of him, that a continuation of the experiment is likely to result in injury, disability, or death to the experimental subject.

Appendix B
World Medical Association Declaration of Helsinki
Recommendations Guiding Physicians in Biomedical Research Involving Human Subjects

Adopted by the 18th World Medical Assembly, Helsinki, Finland, June 1964 and amended by the 29th World Medical Assembly, Tokyo, Japan, October 1975; 35th World Medical Assembly, Venice, Italy, October 1983; 41st World Medical Assembly, Hong Kong, September 1989; and the 48th General Assembly, Somerset West, Republic of South Africa, October 1996

Reprinted with the kind permission of the World Medical Association.

INTRODUCTION

It is the mission of the physician to safeguard the health of the people. His or her knowledge and conscience are dedicated to the fulfillment of this mission.

The Declaration of Geneva of the World Medical Association binds the physician with the words, "The health of my patient will be my first consideration," and the International Code of Medical Ethics declares that, "A physician shall act only in the patient's interest when providing medical care which might have the effect of weakening the physical and mental condition of the patient."

The purpose of biomedical research involving human subjects must be to improve diagnostic, therapeutic and prophylactic procedures and the understanding of the aetiology and pathogenesis of disease.

In current medical practice most diagnostic, therapeutic or prophylactic procedures involve hazards. This applies especially to biomedical research.

Medical progress is based on research which ultimately must rest in part on experimentation involving human subjects.

In the field of biomedical research a fundamental distinction must be recognized between medical research in which the aim is essentially diagnostic or therapeutic for a patient, and medical research, the essential object of which is purely scientific and without implying direct diagnostic or therapeutic value to the person subjected to the research.

Special caution must be exercised in the conduct of research which may affect the environment, and the welfare of animals used for research must be respected.

Because it is essential that the results of laboratory experiments be applied to human beings to further scientific knowledge and to help suffering humanity, the World Medical Association has prepared the following recommendations as a guide to every physician in biomedical research involving human subjects. They should be kept under review in the future. It must be stressed that the standards as drafted are only a guide to physicians all over the world. Physicians are not relieved from criminal, civil and ethical responsibilities under the laws of their own countries.

I. BASIC PRINCIPLES

1. Biomedical research involving human subjects must conform to generally accepted scientific principles and should be based on adequately performed laboratory and animal experimentation and on a thorough knowledge of the scientific literature.
2. The design and performance of each experimental procedure involving human subjects should be clearly formulated in an experimental protocol which should be transmitted for consideration, comment and guidance to a specially appointed committee independent of the investigator and the sponsor provided that this independent committee is in conformity with the laws and regulations of the country in which the research experiment is performed.
3. Biomedical research involving human subjects should be conducted only by scientifically qualified persons and under the supervision of a clinically competent medical person. The responsibility for the human subject must always rest with a medically qualified person and never rest on the subject of the research, even though the subject has given his or her consent.
4. Biomedical research involving human subjects cannot legitimately be carried out unless the importance of the objective is in proportion to the inherent risk to the subject.
5. Every biomedical research project involving human subjects should be preceded by careful assessment of predictable risks in comparison with foreseeable benefits to the subject or to others. Concern for the interests of the subject must always prevail over the interests of science and society.
6. The right of the research subject to safeguard his or her integrity must always be respected. Every precaution should be taken to respect the privacy of the subject and to minimize the impact of the study on the subject's physical and mental integrity and on the personality of the subject.
7. Physicians should abstain from engaging in research projects involving human subjects unless they are satisfied that the hazards involved are believed to be predictable. Physicians should cease any investigation if the hazards are found to outweigh the potential benefits.
8. In publication of the results of his or her research, the physician is obliged to preserve the accuracy of the results. Reports of experimentation not in accordance with the principles laid down in this Declaration should not be accepted for publication.
9. In any research on human beings, each potential subject must be adequately informed of the aims, methods, anticipated benefits and potential hazards of the study and the discomfort it may entail. He or she should be informed that he or she is at liberty to abstain from participation in the study and that he or she is free to withdraw his or her consent to participation at any time. The

physician should then obtain the subject's freely-given informed consent, preferably in writing.

10. When obtaining informed consent for the research project the physician should be particularly cautious if the subject is in a dependent relationship to him or her or may consent under duress. In that case the informed consent should be obtained by a physician who is not engaged in the investigation and who is completely independent of this official relationship.
11. In case of legal incompetence, informed consent should be obtained from the legal guardian in accordance with national legislation. Where physical or mental incapacity makes it impossible to obtain informed consent, or when the subject is a minor, permission from the responsible relative replaces that of the subject in accordance with national legislation.
    Whenever the minor child is in fact able to give a consent, the minor's consent must be obtained in addition to the consent of the minor's legal guardian.
12. The research protocol should always contain a statement of the ethical considerations involved and should indicate that the principles enunciated in the present Declaration are complied with.

II. MEDICAL RESEARCH COMBINED WITH PROFESSIONAL CARE (Clinical Research)

1. In the treatment of the sick person, the physician must be free to use a new diagnostic and therapeutic measure, if in his or her judgment it offers hope of saving life, reestablishing health or alleviating suffering.
2. The potential benefits, hazards and discomfort of a new method should be weighed against the advantages of the best current diagnostic and therapeutic methods.
3. In any medical study, every patient—including those of a control group, if any—should be assured of the best proven diagnostic and therapeutic method. This does not exclude the use of inert placebo in studies where no proven diagnostic or therapeutic method exists.
4. The refusal of the patient to participate in a study must never interfere with the physician-patient relationship.
5. If the physician considers it essential not to obtain informed consent, the specific reasons for this proposal should be stated in the experimental protocol for transmission to the independent committee (I, 2).
6. The physician can combine medical research with professional care, the objective being the acquisition of new medical knowledge, only to the extent that medical research is justified by its potential diagnostic or therapeutic value for the patient.

III. NON-THERAPEUTIC BIOMEDICAL RESEARCH INVOLVING HUMAN SUBJECTS (Non-Clinical Biomedical Research)

1. In the purely scientific application of medical research carried out on a human being, it is the duty of the physician to remain the protector of the life and health of that person on whom biomedical research is being carried out.
2. The subjects should be volunteers—either healthy persons or patients for whom the experimental design is not related to the patient's illness.
3. The investigator or the investigating team should discontinue the research if in his/her or their judgment it may, if continued, be harmful to the individual.

4. In research on man, the interest of science and society should never take precedence over considerations related to the wellbeing of the subject.

Appendix C
The Belmont Report
Ethical Principles and Guidelines for the Protection of Human Subjects of Research

Report of the National Commission for the Protection of Human Subjects of Biomedical and Behavioral Research, Department of Health, Education, and Welfare. 18 April 1979.

Scientific research has produced substantial social benefits. It has also posed some troubling ethical questions. Public attention was drawn to these questions by reported abuses of human subjects in biomedical experiments, especially during the Second World War. During the Nuremberg War Crime Trials, the Nuremberg code was drafted as a set of standards for judging physicians and scientists who had conducted biomedical experiments on concentration camp prisoners. This code became the prototype of many later codes[1] intended to assure that research involving human subjects would be carried out in an ethical manner.

The codes consist of rules, some general, others specific, that guide the investigators or the reviewers of research in their work. Such rules often are inadequate to cover complex situations; at times they come into conflict, and they are frequently difficult to interpret or apply. Broader ethical principles will provide a basis on which specific rules may be formulated, criticized and interpreted.

Three principles, or general prescriptive judgments, that are relevant to research involving human subjects are identified in this statement. Other principles may also be relevant. These three are comprehensive, however, and are stated at a level of generalization that should assist scientists, subjects, reviewers and interested citizens to understand the ethical issues inherent in research involving human subjects. These principles cannot always be applied so as to resolve beyond dispute particular ethical problems. The objective is to provide an analytical framework that will guide the resolution of ethical problems arising from research involving human subjects.

This statement consists of a distinction between research and practice, a discussion of the three basic ethical principles, and remarks about the application of these principles.

A. Boundaries Between Practice and Research

It is important to distinguish between biomedical and behavioral research, on the one hand, and the practice of accepted therapy on the other, in order to know what activities ought to undergo review for the protection of human subjects of research. The distinction between research and practice is blurred partly because both often occur together (as in research designed to evaluate a therapy) and partly because notable departures from standard practice are often called "experimental" when the terms "experimental" and "research" are not carefully defined.

For the most part, the term "practice" refers to interventions that are designed solely to enhance the well being of an individual patient or client and that have a reasonable expectation of success. The purpose of medical or behavioral practice is to provide diagnosis, preventive treatment or therapy to particular individuals.[2] By contrast, the term "research" designates an activity designed to test an hypothesis, permit conclusions to be drawn, and thereby to develop or contribute to generalizable knowledge (expressed, for example, in theories, principles, and statements of relationships). Research is usually described in a formal protocol that sets forth an objective and a set of procedures designed to reach that objective.

When a clinician departs in a significant way from standard or accepted practice, the innovation does not, in and of itself, constitute research. The fact that a procedure is "experimental," in the sense of new, untested or different, does not automatically place it in the category of research. Radically new procedures of this description should, however, be made the object of formal research at an early stage in order to determine whether they are safe and effective. Thus, it is the responsibility of medical practice committees, for example, to insist that a major innovation be incorporated into a formal research project.[3]

Research and practice may be carried on together when research is designed to evaluate the safety and efficacy of a therapy. This need not cause any confusion regarding whether or not the activity requires review; the general rule is that if there is any element of research in an activity, that activity should undergo review for the protection of human subjects.

B. Basic Ethical Principles

The expression "basic ethical principles" refers to those general judgments that serve as a basic justification for the many particular ethical prescriptions and evaluations of human actions. Three basic principles, among those generally accepted in our cultural tradition, are particularly relevant to the ethics of research involving human subjects: The principles of respect for persons, beneficence and justice.

1. Respect for Persons.—Respect for persons incorporates at least two ethical convictions: first, that individuals should be treated as autonomous agents, and second, that persons with diminished autonomy are entitled to protection. The principle of respect for persons thus divides into two separate moral requirements: The requirement to acknowledge autonomy and the requirement to protect those with diminished autonomy.

An autonomous person is an individual capable of deliberation about personal goals and of acting under the direction of such deliberation. To respect autonomy is to give weight to autonomous persons' considered opinions and choices while refraining from obstructing their actions unless they are clearly detrimental to others. To show lack of respect for an autonomous agent is to repudiate that person's considered judgments, to deny an individual the freedom to act on those considered judgments, or to withhold information necessary to make a considered judgment, when there are no compelling reasons to do so.

However, not every human being is capable of self-determination. The capacity for self-determination matures during an individual's life, and some individuals lose this capacity wholly or in part because of illness, mental disability, or circumstances that severely restrict liberty. Respect for the immature and the incapacitated may require protecting them as they mature or while they are incapacitated.

Some persons are in need of extensive protection, even to the point of excluding them from activities which may harm them; other persons require little protection beyond making sure they undertake activities freely and with awareness of possible adverse consequences. The extent of protection afforded should depend upon the risk of harm and the likelihood of benefit. The judgment that any individual lacks autonomy should be periodically reevaluated and will vary in different situations.

In most cases of research involving human subjects, respect for persons demands that subjects enter into the research voluntarily and with adequate information. In some situations, however, application of the principle is not obvious. The involvement of prisoners as subjects of research provides an instructive example. On the one hand, it would seem that the principle of respect for persons requires that prisoners not be deprived of the opportunity to volunteer for research. On the other hand, under prison conditions they may be subtly coerced or unduly influenced to engage in research activities for which they would not otherwise volunteer. Respect for persons would then dictate that prisoners be protected. Whether to allow prisoners to "volunteer" or to "protect" them presents a dilemma. Respecting persons, in most hard cases, is often a matter of balancing competing claims urged by the principle of respect itself.

2. Beneficence.—Persons are treated in an ethical manner not only by respecting their decisions and protecting them from harm, but also by making efforts to secure their well being. Such treatment falls under the principle of beneficence. The term "beneficence" is often understood to cover acts of kindness or charity that go beyond strict obligation. In this document, beneficence is understood in a stronger sense, as an obligation. Two general rules have been formulated as complementary expressions of beneficent actions in this sense: (1) do not harm and (2) maximize possible benefits and minimize possible harms.

The Hippocratic maxim "do no harm" has long been a fundamental principle of medical ethics. Claude Bernard extended it to the realm of research, saying that one should not injure one person regardless of the benefits that might come to others. However, even avoiding harm requires learning what is harmful; and, in the process of obtaining this information, persons may be exposed to risk of harm. Further, the Hippocratic Oath requires physicians to benefit their patients "according to their best judgment." Learning what will in fact benefit may require exposing persons to risk. The problem posed by these imperatives is to decide when it is justifiable to seek certain benefits despite the risks involved, and when the benefits should be foregone because of the risks.

The obligations of beneficence affect both individual investigators and society at large, because they extend both to particular research projects and to the entire enterprise of research. In the case of particular projects, investigators and members of their institutions are obliged to give forethought to the maximization of benefits and the reduction of risk that might occur from the research investigation. In the case of scientific research in general, members of the larger society are obliged to recognize the longer term benefits and risks that may result from the improvement of knowledge and from the development of novel medical, psychotherapeutic, and social procedures.

The principle of beneficence often occupies a well-defined justifying role in many areas of research involving human subjects. An example is found in research involving children. Effective ways of treating childhood diseases and fostering healthy development are benefits that serve to justify research involving children—even when individual research subjects are not direct beneficiaries. Research also makes is possible to avoid the harm that may result from the application of previously accepted routine practices that on closer investigation turn out to be dangerous. But the role of the principle of beneficence is not always so unambiguous. A difficult ethical problem remains, for example, about research that presents more than minimal risk without immediate prospect of direct benefit to the children involved. Some have argued that such research is inadmissible, while others have pointed out that this limit would rule out much research promising great benefit to children in the future. Here again, as with all hard cases, the different claims covered by the principle of beneficence may come into conflict and force difficult choices.

3. Justice.—Who ought to receive the benefits of research and bear its burdens? This is a question of justice, in the sense of "fairness in distribution" or "what is deserved." An injustice occurs when some benefit to which a person is entitled is denied without good reason or when some burden is imposed unduly. Another way of conceiving the principle of justice is that equals ought to be treated equally. However, this statement requires explication. Who is equal and who is unequal? What considerations justify departure from equal distribution? Almost all commentators allow that distinctions based on experience, age, deprivation, competence, merit and position do sometimes constitute criteria justifying differential treatment for certain purposes. It is necessary, then, to explain in what respects people should be treated equally. There are several widely accepted formulations of just ways to distribute burdens and benefits. Each formulation mentions some relevant property on the basis of which burdens and benefits should be distributed. These formulations are (1) to each person an equal share, (2) to each person according to individual need, (3) to each person according to individual effort, (4) to each person according to societal contribution, and (5) to each person according to merit.

Questions of justice have long been associated with social practices such as punishment, taxation and political representation. Until recently these questions have not generally been associated with scientific research. However, they are foreshadowed even in the earliest reflections on the ethics of research involving human subjects. For example, during the 19th and early 20th centuries the burdens of serving as research subjects fell largely upon poor ward patients, while the benefits of improved medical care flowed primarily to private patients. Subsequently, the exploitation of unwilling prisoners as research subjects in Nazi concentration camps was condemned as a particularly flagrant injustice. In this country, in the 1940's, the Tuskegee syphilis study used disadvantaged, rural black men to study the untreated course of a disease that is by no means confined to that population. These subjects were deprived of demonstrably effective treatment in order not to interrupt the project, long after such treatment became generally available.

Against this historical background, it can be seen how conceptions of justice are relevant to research involving human subjects. For example, the selection of research subjects needs to be scrutinized in order to determine whether some classes (e.g., welfare patients, particular racial and ethnic minorities, or persons confined to institutions) are being systematically selected simply because of their easy availability, their compromised position, or their manipulability, rather than for reasons directly related to the problem being studied. Finally, whenever research supported by public funds leads to the development of therapeutic devices and procedures, justice demands both that these not provide advantages only to those who can afford them and that such research should not unduly involve persons from groups unlikely to be among the beneficiaries of subsequent applications of the research.

C. Applications

Applications of the general principles to the conduct of research leads to consideration of the following requirements: Informed consent, risk/benefit assessment, and the selection of subjects of research.

1. Informed Consent.—Respect for persons requires that subjects, to the degree that they are capable, be given the opportunity to choose what shall or shall not happen to them. This opportunity is provided when adequate standards for informed consent are satisfied.

While the importance of informed consent is unquestioned, controversy prevails over the nature and possibility of an informed consent. Nonetheless, there is widespread agreement that the consent process can be analyzed as containing three elements: information, comprehension and voluntariness.

Information. Most codes of research establish specific items for disclosure intended to assure that subjects are given sufficient information. These items generally include: the research procedure, their purposes, risks and anticipated benefits, alternative procedures (where therapy is involved), and a statement offering the subject the opportunity to ask questions and to withdraw at any time from the research. Additional items have been proposed, including how subjects are selected, the person responsible for the research, etc.

However, a simple listing of items does not answer the question of what the standard should be for judging how much and what sort of information should be provided. One standard frequently invoked in medical practice, namely the information commonly provided by practitioners in the field or in the locale, is inadequate since research takes place precisely when a common understanding does not exist. Another standard, currently popular in malpractice law, requires the practitioner to reveal the information that reasonable persons would wish to know in order to make a decision regarding their care. This, too, seems insufficient since the research subject, being in essence a volunteer, may wish to know considerably more about risks gratuitously undertaken than do patients who deliver themselves into the hand of a clinician for needed care. It may be that a standard of "the reasonable volunteer" should be proposed: The extent and nature of information should be such that persons, knowing that the procedure is neither necessary for their care nor perhaps fully understood, can decide whether they wish to participate in the furthering of knowledge. Even when some direct benefit to them is anticipated, the subjects should understand clearly the range of risk and the voluntary nature of participation.

A special problem of consent arises where informing subjects of some pertinent aspect of the research is likely to impair the validity of the research. In many cases, it is sufficient to indicate to subjects that they are being invited to participate in research of which some features will not be revealed until the research is concluded. In all cases of research involving incomplete disclosure, such research is justified only if it is clear that (1) incomplete disclosure is truly necessary to accomplish the goals of the research, (2) there are no undisclosed risks to subjects that are more than minimal, and (3) there is an adequate plan for debriefing subjects, when appropriate, and for dissemination of research results to them. Information about risks should never be withheld for the purpose of eliciting the cooperation of subjects, and truthful answers should always be given to direct questions about the research. Care should be taken to distinguish cases in which disclosure would destroy or invalidate the research from cases in which disclosure would simply inconvenience the investigator.

Comprehension. The manner and context in which information is conveyed is as important as the information itself. For example, presenting information in a disorganized and rapid fashion, allowing too little time for consideration or curtailing opportunities for questioning, all may adversely affect a subject's ability to make an informed choice.

Because the subject's ability to understand is a function of intelligence, rationality, maturity and language, it is necessary to adapt the presentation of the information to the subject's capacities. Investigators are responsible for ascertaining that the subject has comprehended the information. While there is always an obligation to ascertain that the information about risk to subjects is complete and adequately comprehended, when the risks are more serious, that obligation increases. On occasion, it may be suitable to give some oral or written tests of comprehension.

Special provision may need to be made when comprehension is severely limited—for example, by conditions of immaturity or mental disability. Each class of subjects that one might consider as incompetent (e.g., infants and young children, mentally disabled patients, the terminally ill and the comatose) should be considered on its own terms. Even for these persons, however, respect requires giving them the opportunity to choose to the extent they are able, whether or not to participate in research. The objections of these subjects to involvement should be honored, unless the research entails providing them a therapy unavailable elsewhere. Respect for persons also requires seeking the permission of other parties in order to protect the subjects from harm. Such persons are thus respected both by acknowledging their own wishes and by the use of third parties to protect them from harm.

The third parties chosen should be those who are most likely to understand the incompetent subject's situation and to act in that person's best interest. The person authorized to act on behalf of the subject should be given an opportunity to observe the research as it proceeds in order to be able to withdraw the subject from the research, if such action appears in the subject's best interest.

Voluntariness. An agreement to participate in research constitutes a valid consent only if voluntarily given. This element of informed consent requires conditions free of coercion and undue influence. Coercion occurs when an overt threat of harm is intentionally presented by one person to another in order to obtain compliance. Undue influence, by contrast, occurs through an offer of an excessive, unwarranted, inappropriate or improper reward or other overture in order to obtain compliance. Also, inducements that would ordinarily be acceptable may become undue influences if the subject is especially vulnerable.

Unjustifiable pressures usually occur when persons in positions of authority or commanding influence—especially where possible sanctions are involved—urge a course of action for a subject. A continuum of such influencing factors exists, however, and it is impossible to state precisely where justifiable persuasion ends and undue influence begins. But undue influence would include actions such as manipulating a person's choice through the controlling influence of a close relative and threatening to withdraw health services to which an individual would otherwise be entitled.

2. Assessment of Risks and Benefits.—The assessment of risks and benefits requires a careful arrayal of relevant data, including, in some cases, alternative ways of obtaining the benefits sought in the research. Thus, the assessment presents both an opportunity and a responsibility to gather systematic and comprehensive information about proposed research. For the investigator, it is a means to examine whether the proposed research is properly designed. For a review committee, it is a method for determining whether the risks that will be presented to subjects are justified. For prospective subjects, the assessment will assist the determination whether or not to participate.

The Nature and Scope of Risks and Benefits. The requirement that research be justified on the basis of a favorable risk/benefit assessment bears a close relation to the principle of beneficence, just as the moral requirement that informed consent be obtained is derived primarily from the principle of respect for persons. The term "risk" refers to a possibility that harm may occur. However, when expressions such as "small risk" or "high risk" are used, they usually refer (often ambiguously) both to the chance (probability) of experiencing a harm and the severity (magnitude) of the envisioned harm.

The term "benefit" is used in the research context to refer to something of positive value related to health or welfare. Unlike "risk," "benefit" is not a term that expresses probabilities. Risk is properly contrasted to probability of benefits, and benefits are properly contrasted with harms rather than risks of harm. Accordingly, so-called risk benefit assessments are concerned with the probabilities and magnitudes of possible harms and anticipated benefits. Many kinds of possible harms and benefits need to be taken into account. There are, for example, risks of psychological harm, physical harm, legal harm, social harm and economic harm and the corresponding benefits. While the most likely types of harms to research subjects are those of psychological or physical pain or injury, other possible kinds should not be overlooked.

Risks and benefits of research may affect the individual subjects, the families of the individual subjects, and society at large (or special groups of subjects in society). Previous codes and Federal regulations have required that risks to subjects be outweighed by the sum of both the anticipated benefit to the subject, if any, and the anticipated benefit to society in the form of knowledge to be gained from the research. In balancing these different elements, the risks and benefits affecting the immediate research subject will normally carry special weight. On the other hand, interests other than those of the subject may on some occasions be sufficient by themselves to justify the risks involved in the research, so long as the subjects' rights have been protected. Beneficence thus requires that we protect against risk of harm to subjects and also that we be concerned about the loss of the substantial benefits that might be gained from research.

The Systematic Assessment of Risks and Benefits. It is commonly said that benefits and risks must be "balanced" and shown to be "in a favorable ratio." The metaphorical character of these terms draws attention to the difficulty of making precise judgments. Only on rare occasions will quantitative techniques be available for the scrutiny of research protocols. However, the idea of systematic, nonarbitrary analysis of risks and benefits should be emulated insofar as possible. This ideal requires those making decisions about the justifiability of research to be thorough in the accumulation and assessment of information about all aspects of the research, and to consider alternatives systematically. This procedure renders the assessment of research more rigorous and precise, while making communication between review board members and investigators less subject to misinterpretation, misinformation and conflicting judgments. Thus, there should first be a determination of the validity of the presuppositions of the research; then the nature, probability and magnitude of risk should be distinguished with as much clarity as possible. The method of ascertaining risks should be explicit, especially where there is no alternative to the use of such vague categories as small or slight risk. It should also be determined whether an investigator's estimates of the probability of harm or benefits are reasonable, as judged by known facts or other available studies.

Finally, assessment of the justifiability of research should reflect at least the following considerations: (i) Brutal or inhumane treatment of human subjects is never morally justified; (ii) Risks should be reduced to those necessary to achieve the research objective. It should be determined whether it is in fact necessary to use human subjects at all. Risk can perhaps never be entirely eliminated, but it can often be reduced by careful attention to alternative procedures; (iii) When research involves significant risk of serious impairment, review committees should be extraordinarily insistent on the justification of the risk (looking usually to the likelihood of benefit to the subject or, in some rare cases, to the manifest voluntariness of the participation); (iv) When vulnerable populations are involved in research, the appropriateness of involving them should itself be demonstrated. A number of variables go into such judgments, including the nature and degree of risk, the condition of the particular population involved, and the nature and level of the anticipated benefits; and (v) Relevant risks and benefits must be thoroughly arrayed in documents and procedures used in the informed consent process.

3. Selection of Subjects.—Just as the principle of respect for persons finds expression in the requirements for consent, and the principle of beneficence in risk/benefit assessment, the principle of justice gives rise to moral requirements that there be fair procedures and outcomes in the selection of research subjects.

Justice is relevant to the selection of subjects of research at two levels: the social and the individual. Individual justice in the selection of subjects would require that researchers exhibit fairness: Thus, they should not offer potentially beneficial research only to some patients who are in their favor or select only "undesirable" persons for risky research. Social justice requires that distinction be drawn between classes of subjects that ought, and ought not, to participate in any particular kind of research, based on the ability of members of that class to bear burdens and on the appropriateness of placing further burdens on already burdened persons. Thus, it can be considered a matter of social justice that there is an order of preference in the selection of classes of subjects (e.g., adults before children) and that some classes of potential subjects (e.g., the institutionalized mentally infirm or prisoners) may be involved as research subjects, if at all, only on certain conditions.

Injustice may appear in the selection of subjects, even if individual subjects are selected fairly by investigators and treated fairly in the course of research. Thus injustice arises from social, racial, sexual and cultural biases institutionalized in society. Thus, even if individual researchers are treating their research subjects fairly, and even if IRBs are taking care to assure that subjects are selected fairly within a particular institution, unjust social patterns may nevertheless appear in the overall distribution of the burdens and benefits of research. Although individual institutions or investigators may not be able to resolve a problem that is pervasive in their social setting, they can consider distributive justice in selecting research subjects.

Some populations, especially institutionalized ones, are already burdened in many ways by their infirmities and environments. When research is proposed that involves risks and does not include a therapeutic component, other less burdened classes of persons should be called upon first to accept these risks of research, except where the research is directly related to the specific conditions of the class involved. Also, even though public funds for research may often flow in the same directions as public funds for health care, it seems unfair that populations dependent on public health care constitute a pool of preferred research subjects if more advantaged populations are likely to be the recipients of the benefits.

One special instance of injustice results from the involvement of vulnerable subjects. Certain groups, such as racial minorities, the economically disadvantaged, the very sick, and the institutionalized may continually be sought as research subjects, owing to their ready availability in settings where research is conducted. Given their dependent status and their frequently compromised capacity for free consent, they should be protected against the danger of being involved in research solely for administrative convenience, or because they are easy to manipulate as a result of their illness or socioeconomic condition.

NOTES

1. Since 1945, various codes for the proper and responsible conduct of human experimentation in medical research have been adopted by different organizations. The best known of these codes are the Nuremberg Code of 1948, the Helsinki Declaration of 1964 (revised in 1975), and the 1971 Guidelines (codified into Federal Regulations in 1974) issued by the U.S. Department of Health, Education, and Welfare Codes for the conduct of social and behavioral research have also been adopted, the best known being that of the American Psychological Association, published in 1973.

2. Although practice usually involves interventions designed solely to enhance the well being of a particular individual, interventions are sometimes applied to one individual for the enhancement of the well-being of another (e.g., blood donation, skin grafts, organ transplants) or an intervention may have the dual purpose of enhancing the well-being of a particular individual, and, at the same time, providing some benefit to others (e.g., vaccination, which pro-

tects both the person who is vaccinated and society generally). The fact that some forms of practice have elements other than immediate benefit to the individual receiving an intervention, however, should not confuse the general distinction between research and practice. Even when a procedure applied in practice may benefit some other person, it remains an intervention designed to enhance the well-being of a particular individual or groups of individuals; thus, it is practice and need not be reviewed as research.

3. Because the problems related to social experimentation may differ substantially from those of biomedical and behavioral research, the Commission specifically declines to make any policy determination regarding such research at this time. Rather, the Commission believes that the problem ought to be addressed by one of its successor bodies.

Appendix D
The "Common Rule"

56 Federal Register *28012. 18 June 1991.*

§__.101 To what does this policy apply?

(a) Except as provided in paragraph (b) of this section, this policy applies to all research involving human subjects conducted, supported or otherwise subject to regulation by any federal department or agency which takes appropriate administrative action to make the policy applicable to such research. This includes research conducted by federal civilian employees or military personnel, except that each department or agency head may adopt such procedural modifications as may be appropriate from an administrative standpoint. It also includes research conducted, supported, or otherwise subject to regulation by the federal government outside the United States.

(1) Research that is conducted or supported by a federal department or agency, whether or not it is regulated as defined in §__.102(e), must comply with all sections of this policy.

(2) Research that is neither conducted nor supported by a federal department or agency but is subject to regulation as defined in §__.102(e) must be reviewed and approved, in compliance with §__.101, §__.102, and §__.107 through §__.117 of this policy, by an institutional review board (IRB) that operates in accordance with the pertinent requirements of this policy.

(b) Unless otherwise required by department or agency heads, research activities in which the only involvement of human subjects will be in one or more of the following categories are exempt from this policy:

(1) Research conducted in established or commonly accepted educational settings, involving normal educational practices, such as: (i) research on regular and special education instructional strategies; or (ii) research on the effectiveness of or the comparison among instructional techniques, curricula, or classroom management methods.

(2) Research involving the use of educational tests (cognitive, diagnostic, aptitude, achievement), survey procedures, interview procedures or observation of public behavior, unless:

(i) Information obtained is recorded in such a manner that human subjects can be identified, directly or through identifiers linked to the subjects; and (ii) any disclosure of the human subjects' responses outside the research could reasonably place the subjects at risk of criminal or civil liability or be damaging to the subjects' financial standing, employability, or reputation.

(3) Research involving the use of educational tests (cognitive, diagnostic, aptitude, achievement), survey procedures, interview procedures, or observation of public behavior that is not exempt under paragraph (b)(2) of this section, if: (i) The human subjects are elected or appointed public officials or candidates for public office; or (ii) federal statute(s) require(s) without exception that the confidentiality of the personally identifiable information will be maintained throughout the research and thereafter.

(4) Research, involving the collection or study of existing data, documents, records, pathological specimens, or diagnostic specimens, if these sources are publicly available or if the information is recorded by the investigator in such a manner that subjects cannot be identified, directly or through identifiers linked to the subjects.

(5) Research and demonstration projects which are conducted by or subject to the approval of department of agency heads, and which are designed to study, evaluate, or otherwise examine: (i) Public benefit or service programs; (ii) procedures for obtaining benefits or services under those programs; (iii) possible changes in or alternatives to those programs or procedures; or (iv) possible changes in methods or levels of payment for benefits or services under those programs.

(6) Taste and food quality evaluation and consumer acceptance studies; (i) if wholesome foods without additives are consumed; or (ii) if a food is consumed that contains a food ingredient at or below the level and for a use found to be safe, or agricultural chemical or environmental contaminant at or below the level found to be safe, by the Food and Drug Administration or approved by the Environmental Protection Agency or the Food Safety and Inspection Service of the U.S. Department of Agriculture.

(c) Department or agency heads retain final judgment as to whether a particular activity is covered by this policy.

(d) Department or agency heads may require that specific research activities or classes of research activities conducted, supported, or otherwise subject to regulation by the department or agency but not otherwise covered by this policy, comply with some or all of the requirements of this policy.

(e) Compliance with this policy requires compliance with pertinent federal laws or regulations which provide additional protections for human subjects.

(f) This policy does not affect any state or local laws or regulations which may otherwise be applicable and which provide additional protections for human subjects.

(g) This policy does not affect any foreign laws or regulations which may otherwise be applicable and which provide additional protections to human subjects of research.

(h) When research covered by this policy takes place in foreign countries, procedures normally followed in the foreign countries to protect human subjects may differ from those set forth in this policy. [An example is a foreign institution which complies with guidelines consistent with the World Medical Assembly Declaration (Declaration of Helsinki amended 1989) issued either by sovereign states or by an organization whose function for the protection of human research subjects is internationally recognized.] In these circumstances, if a department or agency head determines that the procedures prescribed by the institution afford protections that are at least equivalent to those provided in this policy, the department or agency head may approve the substitution of the foreign procedures in lieu of the procedural requirements provided in this policy. Except when otherwise required by statute, Executive Order, or the department or agency head, notices of these actions as they occur will be published in the **Federal Register** or will be otherwise published as provided in department or agency procedures.

(i) Unless otherwise required by law, department or agency heads may waive the applicability of some or all of the provisions of this policy to specific research activities or classes of research activities otherwise covered by this policy. Except when otherwise required by statute or Executive Order, the department or agency head shall forward advance notices of these actions to the Office for Protection from Research Risks, Department of Health and Human Services (HHS), and shall also publish them in the **Federal Register** or in such a manner as provided in department or agency procedures. Institutions with HHS-approved assurances on file will abide by provisions of title 45 CFR part 46 subparts A-D. Some of the other Departments and Agencies have incorporated all provisions of title 45 CFR part 46 into their policies and procedures as well. However, the exemptions at 45 CFR part 46.101(b) do not apply to research involving prisoners, fetuses, pregnant women, or human in vitro fertilization, subparts B and C. The exemption at 45 CFR part 46.101(b)(2), for research involving survey or interview procedures or observation of public behavior, does not apply to research with children, subpart D, except for research involving observations of public behavior when the investigator(s) do not participate in the activities being observed.

§ __.102 Definitions.

(a) *Department or agency head* means the head of any federal department or agency and any other officer or employee of any department or agency to whom authority has been delegated.

(b) *Institution* means any public or private entity or agency (including federal, state, and other agencies).

(c) *Legally authorized representative* means an individual or judicial or other body authorized under applicable law to consent on behalf of a prospective subject to the subject's participation in the procedure(s) involved in the research.

(d) *Research* means a systematic investigation, including research development, testing and evaluation, designed to develop or contribute to generalizable knowledge. Activities which meet this definition constitute research for purposes of this policy, whether or not they are conducted or supported under a program which is considered research for other purposes. For example, some demonstration and service programs may include research activities.

(e) *Research subject to regulation*, and similar terms are intended to encompass those research activities for which a federal department or agency has specific responsibility for regulating as a research activity, (for example, Investigational New Drug requirements administered by the Food and Drug Administration). It does not include research activities which are incidentally regulated by a federal department or agency solely as part of the department's or agency's broader responsibility to regulate certain types of activities whether research or non-research in nature (for example, Wage and Hour requirements administered by the Department of Labor).

(f) *Human subject* means a living individual about whom an investigator (whether professional or student) conducting research obtains (1) data through intervention or interaction with the individual, or

(2) identifiable private information. Intervention includes both physical procedures by which data are gathered (for example, venipuncture) and manipulations of the subject or the subject's environment that are performed for research purposes. Interaction includes communication or interpersonal contact between investigator and subject. "Private information" includes information about behavior that occurs in a context in which an individual can reasonably expect that no observation or recording is taking place, and information which has been provided for specific purposes by an individual and which the individual can reasonably expect will not be made public (for example, a medical record). Private information must be individually identifiable (i.e., the identity of the subject is or may readily be ascertained by the investigator or associated with the information) in order for obtaining the information to constitute research involving human subjects.

(g) *IRB* means an institutional review board established in accord with and for the purposes expressed in this policy.

(h) *IRB approval* means the determination of the IRB that the research has been reviewed and may be conducted at an institution within the constraints set forth by the IRB and by other institutional and federal requirements.

(i) *Minimal risk* means that the probability and magnitude of harm or discomfort anticipated in the research are not greater in and of themselves than those ordinarily encountered in daily life or during the performance of routine physical or psychological examinations or tests.

(j) *Certification* means the official notification by the institution to the supporting department or agency, in accordance with the requirements of this policy, that a research project or activity involving human subjects has been reviewed and approved by an IRB in accordance with an approved assurance.

§ __.103 Assuring compliance with this policy—research conducted or supported by any Federal Department or Agency.

(a) Each institution engaged in research which is covered by this policy and which is conducted or supported by a federal department or agency shall provide written assurance satisfactory to the department or agency head that it will comply with the requirements set forth in this policy. In lieu of requiring submission of an assurance, individual department or agency heads shall accept the existence of a current assurance, appropriate for the research in question, on file with the Office for Protection from Research Risks, HHS, and approved for Federalwide use by that office. When the existence of an HHS-approved assurance is accepted in lieu of requiring submission of an assurance, reports (except certification) required by this policy to be made to department and agency heads shall also be made to the Office for Protection from Research Risks, HHS.

(b) Departments and agencies will conduct or support research covered by this policy only if the institution has an assurance approved as provided in this section, and only if the institution has certified to the department or agency head that the research has been reviewed and approved by an IRB provided for in the assurance, and will be subject to continuing review by the IRB. Assurances applicable to federally supported or conducted research shall at a minimum include:

(1) A statement of principles governing the institution in the discharge of its responsibilities for protecting the rights and welfare of human subjects of research conducted at or sponsored by the institution, regardless of whether the research is subject to federal regulation. This may include an appropriate existing code, declaration, or statement of ethical principles, or a statement formulated by the institution itself. This requirement does not preempt provi-

sions of this policy applicable to department- or agency-supported or regulated research and need not be applicable to any research exempted or waived under §__.101 (b) or (i).

(2) Designation of one or more IRBs established in accordance with the requirements of this policy, and for which provisions are made for meeting space and sufficient staff to support the IRB's review and recordkeeping duties.

(3) A list of IRB members identified by name; earned degrees; representative capacity; indications of experience such as board certifications, licenses, etc., sufficient to describe each member's chief anticipated contributions to IRB deliberations; and any employment or other relationship between each member and the institution; for example: full-time employee, part-time employee, member of governing panel or board, stockholder, paid or unpaid consultant. Changes in IRB membership shall be reported to the department or agency head, unless in accord with §__.103(a) of this policy, the existence of an HHS-approved assurance is accepted. In this case, change in IRB membership shall be reported to the Office for Protection from Research Risks, HHS.

(4) Written procedures which the IRB will follow: (i) for conducting its initial and continuing review of research and for reporting its findings and actions to the investigator and the institution; (ii) for determining which projects require review more often than annually and which projects need verification from sources other than the investigators that no material changes have occurred since previous IRB review; and (iii) for ensuring prompt reporting to the IRB of proposed changes in a research activity, and for ensuring that such changes in approved research, during the period for which IRB approval has already been given, may not be initiated without IRB review and approval except when necessary to eliminate apparent immediate hazards to the subject.

(5) Written procedures for ensuring prompt reporting to the IRB, appropriate institutional officials, and the department or agency head of: (i) any unanticipated problems involving risks to subjects or others or any serious or continuing noncompliance with this policy or the requirements or determinations of the IRB; and (ii) any suspension or termination of IRB approval.

(c) The assurance shall be executed by an individual authorized to act for the institution and to assume on behalf of the institution the obligations imposed by this policy and shall be filed in such form and manner as the department or agency head prescribes.

(d) The department or agency head will evaluate all assurances submitted in accordance with this policy through such officers and employees of the department or agency and such experts or consultants engaged for this purpose as the department or agency head determines to be appropriate. The department or agency head's evaluation will take into consideration the adequacy of the proposed IRB in light of the anticipated scope of the institution's research activities and the types of subject populations likely to be involved, the appropriateness of the proposed initial and continuing review procedures in light of the probable risks, and the size and complexity of the institution.

(e) On the basis of this evaluation, the department or agency head may approve or disapprove the assurance, or enter into negotiations to develop an approvable one. The department or agency head may limit the period during which any particular approved assurance or class of approved assurances shall remain effective or otherwise condition or restrict approval.

(f) Certification is required when the research is supported by a federal department or agency and not otherwise exempted or waived under §__.101 (b) or (i). An institution with an approved assurance shall certify that each application or proposal for research covered by the assurance and by §__.103 of this Policy has been reviewed and approved by the IRB. Such certification must be submitted with the application or proposal or by such later date as may be prescribed by the department or agency to which the application or proposal is submitted. Under no condition shall research covered by §__.103 of the Policy be supported prior to receipt of the certification that the research has been reviewed and approved by the IRB. Institutions without an approved assurance covering the research shall certify within 30 days after receipt of a request for such a certification from the department or agency, that the application or proposal has been approved by the IRB. If the certification is not submitted within these time limits, the application or proposal may be returned to the institution. (Approved by the Office of Management and Budget under Control Number 9999-0020.)

§__.104-106 [Reserved]

§__.107 IRB membership.

(a) Each IRB shall have at least five members, with varying backgrounds to promote complete and adequate review of research activities commonly conducted by the institution. The IRB shall be sufficiently qualified through the experience and expertise of its members, and the diversity of the members, including consideration of race, gender, and cultural backgrounds and sensitivity to such issues as community attitudes, to promote respect for its advice and counsel in safeguarding the rights and welfare of human subjects. In addition to possessing the professional competence necessary to review specific research activities, the IRB shall be able to ascertain the acceptability of proposed research in terms of institutional commitments and regulations, applicable law, and standards of professional conduct and practice. The IRB shall therefore include persons knowledgeable in these areas. If an IRB regularly reviews research that involves a vulnerable category of subjects, such as children, prisoners, pregnant women, or handicapped or mentally disabled persons, consideration shall be given to the inclusion of one or more individuals who are knowledgeable about and experienced in working with these subjects.

(b) Every nondiscriminatory effort will be made to ensure that no IRB consists entirely of men or entirely of women, including the institution's consideration of qualified persons of both sexes, so long as no selection is made to the IRB on the basis of gender. No IRB may consist entirely of members of one profession.

(c) Each IRB shall include at least one member whose primary concerns are in scientific areas and at least one member whose primary concerns are in nonscientific areas.

(d) Each IRB shall include at least one member who is not otherwise affiliated with the institution and who is not part of the immediate family of a person who is affiliated with the institution.

(e) No IRB may have a member participate in the IRB's initial or continuing review of any project in which the member has a conflicting interest, except to provide information requested by the IRB.

(f) An IRB may, in its discretion, invite individuals with competence in special areas to assist in the review of issues which require expertise beyond or in addition to that available on the IRB. These individuals may not vote with the IRB.

§__.108 IRB functions and operations.

In order to fulfill the requirements of this policy each IRB shall:

(a) Follow written procedures in the

same detail as described in §__.103(b)(4) and, to the extent required by, §__.103(b)(5).

(b) Except when an expedited review procedure is used (see §__.110), review proposed research at convened meetings at which a majority of the members of the IRB are present, including at least one member whose primary concerns are in nonscientific areas. In order for the research to be approved, it shall receive the approval of a majority of those members present at the meeting.

§__.109 IRB review of research.

(a) An IRB shall review and have authority to approve, require modifications in (to secure approval), or disapprove all research activities covered by this policy.

(b) An IRB shall require that information given to subjects as part of informed consent is in accordance with §__.116. The IRB may require that information, in addition to that specifically mentioned in §__.116, be given to the subjects when in the IRB's judgment the information would meaningfully add to the protection of the rights and welfare of subjects.

(c) An IRB shall require documentation of informed consent or may waive documentation in accordance with §__.117.

(d) An IRB shall notify investigators and the institution in writing of its decision to approve or disapprove the proposed research activity, or of modifications required to secure IRB approval of the research activity. If the IRB decides to disapprove a research activity, it shall include in its written notification a statement of the reasons for its decision and give the investigator an opportunity to respond in person or in writing.

(e) An IRB shall conduct continuing review of research covered by this policy at intervals appropriate to the degree of risk, but not less than once per year, and shall have authority to observe or have a third party observe the consent process and the research. (Approved by the Office of Management and Budget under Control Number 9999-0020.)

§__.110 Expedited review procedures for certain kinds of research involving no more than minimal risk, and for minor changes in approved research.

(a) The Secretary, HHS, has established, and published as a Notice in the **Federal Register**, a list of categories of research that may be reviewed by the IRB through an expedited review procedure. The list will be amended, as appropriate after consultation with other departments and agencies, through periodic republication by the Secretary, HHS, in the **Federal Register**. A copy of the list is available from the Office for Protection from Research Risks, National Institutes of Health, HHS, Bethesda, Maryland 20892.

(b) An IRB may use the expedited review procedure to review either or both of the following:

(1) Some or all of the research appearing on the list and found by the reviewer(s) to involve no more than minimal risk,

(2) Minor changes in previously approved research during the period (of one year or less) for which approval is authorized. Under an expedited review procedure, the review may be carried out by the IRB chairperson or by one or more experienced reviewers designated by the chairperson from among members of the IRB. In reviewing the research, the reviewers may exercise all of the authorities of the IRB except that the reviewers may not disapprove the research. A research activity may be disapproved only after review in accordance with the non-expedited procedure set forth in §__.108(b).

(c) Each IRB which uses an expedited review procedure shall adopt a method for keeping all members advised of research proposals which have been approved under the procedure.

(d) The department or agency head may restrict, suspend, terminate, or choose not to authorize an institution's or IRB's use of the expedited review procedure.

§__.111 Criteria for IRB approval of research.

(a) In order to approve research covered by this policy the IRB shall determine that all of the following requirements are satisfied:

(1) Risks to subjects are minimized: (i) By usmng procedures which are consistent with sound research design and which do not unnecessarily expose subjects to risk; and (ii) whenever appropriate, by using procedures already being performed on the subjects for diagnostic or treatment purposes.

(2) Risks to subjects are reasonable in relation to anticipated benefits, if any, to subjects, and the importance of the knowledge that may reasonably be expected to result. In evaluating risks and benefits, the IRB should consider only those risks and benefits that may result from the research (as distinguished from risks and benefits of therapies subjects would receive even if not participating in the research). The IRB should not consider possible long-range effects of applying knowledge gained in the research (for example, the possible effects of the research on public policy) as among those research risks that fall within the purview of its responsibility.

(3) Selection of subjects is equitable. In making this assessment the IRB should take into account the purposes of the research and the setting in which the research will be conducted and should be particularly cognizant of the special problems of research involving vulnerable populations, such as children, prisoners, pregnant women, mentally disabled persons, or economically or educationally disadvantaged persons.

(4) Informed consent will be sought from each prospective subject or the subject's legally authorized representative, in accordance with, and to the extent required by §__.116.

(5) Informed consent will be appropriately documented, in accordance with, and to the extent required by §__.117.

(6) When appropriate, the research plan makes adequate provision for monitoring the data collected to ensure the safety of subjects.

(7) When appropriate, there are adequate provisions to protect the privacy of subjects and to maintain the confidentiality of data.

(b) When some or all of the subjects are likely to be vulnerable to coercion or undue influence, such as children, prisoners, pregnant women, mentally disabled persons, or economically or educationally disadvantaged persons, additional safeguards have been included in the study to protect the rights and welfare of these subjects.

§__.112 Review by institution.

Research covered by this policy that has been approved by an IRB may be subject to further appropriate review and approval or disapproval by officials of the institution. However, those officials may not approve the research if it has not been approved by an IRB.

§__.113 Suspension or termination of IRB approval of research.

An IRB shall have authority to suspend or terminate approval of research that is not being conducted in accordance with the IRB's requirements or that has been associated with unexpected serious harm to subjects. Any suspension or termination of approval shall include a statement of the reasons for the IRB's action and shall be reported promptly to the investigator, appropriate institutional officials, and the department or agency head. (Approved by the Office of Management and Budget under Control Number 9999-0020.)

§__.114 Cooperative research.

Cooperative research projects are those projects covered by this policy which involve more than one institution. In the conduct of cooperative research projects, each institution is responsible for safeguarding the rights and welfare of human subjects and for complying with this policy. With the approval of the department or agency head, an institution participating in a cooperative project may enter into a joint review arrangement, rely upon the review of another qualified IRB, or make similar arrangements for avoiding duplication of effort.

§__.115 IRB records.

(a) An institution, or when appropriate an IRB, shall prepare and maintain adequate documentation of IRB activities, including the following:

(1) Copies of all research proposals reviewed, scientific evaluations, if any, that accompany the proposals, approved sample consent documents, progress reports submitted by investigators, and reports of injuries to subjects.

(2) Minutes of IRB meetings which shall be in sufficient detail to show attendance at the meetings; actions taken by the IRB; the vote on these actions including the number of members voting for, against, and abstaining; the basis for requiring changes in or disapproving research; and a written summary of the discussion of controverted issues and their resolution.

(3) Records of continuing review activities.

(4) Copies of all correspondence between the IRB and the investigators.

(5) A list of IRB members in the same detail as described is §__.103(b)(3).

(6) Written procedures for the IRB in the same detail as described in §__.103(b)(4) and §__.103(b)(5).

(7) Statements of significant new findings provided to subjects, as required by §__.116(b)(5).

(b) The records required by this policy shall be retained for at least 3 years, and records relating to research which is conducted shall be retained for at least 3 years after completion of the research. All records shall be accessible for inspection and copying by authorized representatives of the department or agency at reasonable times and in a reasonable manner. (Approved by the Office of Management and Budget under Control Number 9999-0020.)

§__.116 General requirements for informed consent.

Except as provided elsewhere in this policy, no investigator may involve a human being as a subject in research covered by this policy unless the investigator has obtained the legally effective informed consent of the subject or the subject's legally authorized representative. An investigator shall seek such consent only under circumstances that provide the prospective subject or the representative sufficient opportunity to consider whether or not to participate and that minimize the possibility of coercion or undue influence. The information that is given to the subject or the representative shall be in language understandable to the subject or the representative. No informed consent, whether oral or written, may include any exculpatory language through which the subject or the representative is made to waive or appear to waive any of the subject's legal rights, or releases or appears to release the investigator, the sponsor, the institution or its agents from liability for negligence.

(a) Basic elements of informed consent.

Except as provided in paragraph (c) or (d) of this section, in seeking informed consent the following information shall be provided to each subject:

(1) A statement that the study involves research, an explanation of the purposes of the research and the expected duration of the subject's participation, a description of the procedures to be followed, and identification of any procedures which are experimental;

(2) A description of any reasonably foreseeable risks or discomforts to the subject;

(3) A description of any benefits to the subject or to others which may reasonably be expected from the research;

(4) A disclosure of appropriate alternative procedures or courses of treatment, if any, that might be advantageous to the subject;

(5) A statement describing the extent, if any, to which confidentiality of records identifying the subject will be maintained;

(6) For research involving more than minimal risk, an explanation as to whether any compensation and an explanation as to whether any medical treatments are available if injury occurs and, if so, what they consist of, or where further information may be obtained;

(7) An explanation of whom to contact for answers to pertinent questions about the research and research subjects' rights, and whom to contact in the event of a research-related injury to the subject; and

(8) A statement that participation is voluntary, refusal to participate will involve no penalty or loss of benefits to which the subject is otherwise entitled, and the subject may discontinue participation at any time without penalty or loss of benefits to which the subject is otherwise entitled.

(b) Additional elements of informed consent. When appropriate, one or more of the following elements of information shall also be provided to each subject:

(1) A statement that the particular treatment or procedure may involve risks to the subject (or to the embryo or fetus, if the subject is or may become pregnant) which are currently unforeseeable;

(2) Anticipated circumstances under which the subject's participation may be terminated by the investigator without regard to the subject's consent;

(3) Any additional costs to the subject that may result from participation in the research;

(4) The consequences of a subject's decision to withdraw from the research and procedures for orderly termination of participation by the subject;

(5) A statement that significant new findings developed during the course of the research which may relate to the subject's willingness to continue participation will be provided to the subject; and

(6) The approximate number of subjects involved in the study.

(c) An IRB may approve a consent procedure which does not include, or which alters, some or all of the elements of informed consent set forth above, or waive the requirement to obtain informed consent provided the IRB finds and documents that:

(1) The research or demonstration project is to be conducted by or subject to the approval of state or local government officials and is designed to study, evaluate, or otherwise examine: (i) Public benefit of service programs; (ii) procedures for obtaining benefits or services under those programs; (iii) possible changes in or alternatives to those programs or procedures; or (iv) possible changes in methods or levels of payment for benefits or services under those programs; and

(2) The research could not practicably be carried out without the waiver or

alteration.

(d) An IRB may approve a consent procedure which does not include, or which alters, some or all of the elements of informed consent set forth in this section, or waive the requirements to obtain informed consent provided the IRB finds and documents that:

(1) The research involves no more than minimal risk to the subjects;

(2) The waiver or alteration will not adversely affect the rights and welfare of the subjects;

(3) The research could not practicably be carried out without the waiver or alteration; and

(4) Whenever appropriate, the subjects will be provided with additional pertinent information after participation.

(e) The informed consent requirements in this policy are not intended to preempt any applicable federal, state, or local laws which require additional information to be disclosed in order for informed consent to be legally effective.

(f) Nothing in this policy is intended to limit the authority of a physician to provide emergency medical care, to the extent the physician is permitted to do so under applicable federal, state, or local law. (Approved by the Office of Management and Budget under Control Number 9999-0020.)

§__.117 Documentation of informed consent.

(a) Except as provided in paragraph (c) of this section, informed consent shall be documented by the use of a written consent form approved by the IRB and signed by the subject or the subject's legally authorized representative. A copy shall be given to the person signing the form.

(b) Except as provided in paragraph (c) of this section, the consent form may be either of the following:

(1) A written consent document that embodies the elements of informed consent required by §__.116. This form may be read to the subject or the subject's legally authorized representative, but in any event, the investigator shall give either the subject or the representative adequate opportunity to read it before it is signed; or

(2) A short form written consent document stating that the elements of informed consent required by §__.116 have been presented orally to the subject or the subject's legally authorized representative. When this method is used, there shall be a witness to the oral presentation. Also, the IRB shall approve a written summary of what is to be said to the subject or the representative. Only the short form itself is to be signed by the subject or the representative. However, the witness shall sign both the short form and a copy of the summary, and the person actually obtaining consent shall sign a copy of the summary. A copy of the summary shall be given to the subject or the representative, in addition to a copy of the short form.

(c) An IRB may waive the requirement for the investigator to obtain a signed consent form for some or all subjects if it finds either:

(1) That the only record linking the subject and the research would be the consent document and the principal risk would be potential harm resulting from a breach of confidentiality. Each subject will be asked whether the subject wants documentation linking the subject with the research, and the subject's wishes will govern; or

(2) That the research presents no more than minimal risk of harm to subjects and involves no procedures for which written consent is normally required outside of the research context. In cases in which the documentation requirement is waived, the IRB may require the investigator to provide subjects with a written statement regarding the research. (Approved by

the Office of Management and Budget under Control Number 9999-0020.)

§__.118 Applications and proposals lacking definite plans for involvement of human subjects.

Certain types of applications for grants, cooperative agreements, or contracts are submitted to departments or agencies with the knowledge that subjects may be involved within the period of support, but definite plans would not normally be set forth in the application or proposal. These include activities such as institutional type grants when selection of specific projects is the institution's responsibility; research training grants in which the activities involving subjects remain to be selected; and projects in which human subject's involvement will depend upon completion of instruments, prior animal studies, or purification of compounds. These applications need not be reviewed by an IRB before an award may be made. However, except for research exempted or waived under §__.101 (b) or (i), no human subjects may be involved in any project supported by these awards until the project has been reviewed and approved by the IRB, as provided in this policy, and certification submitted, by the institution, to the department or agency.

§__.119 Research undertaken without the intention of involving human subjects.

In the event research is undertaken without the intention of involving human subjects, but it is later proposed to involve human subjects in the research, the research shall first be reviewed and approved by an IRB, as provided in this policy, a certification submitted, by the institution, to the department or agency, and final approval given to the proposed change by the department or agency.

§__.120 Evaluation and disposition of applications and proposals for research to be conducted or supported by a Federal Department or Agency.

(a) The department or agency head will evaluate all applications and proposals involving human subjects submitted to the department or agency through such officers and employees of the department or agency and such experts and consultants as the department or agency head determines to be appropriate. This evaluation will take into consideration the risks to the subjects, the adequacy of protection against these risks, the potential benefits of the research to the subjects and others, and the importance of the knowledge gained or to be gained.

(b) On the basis of this evaluation, the department or agency head may approve or disapprove the application or proposal, or enter into negotiations to develop an approvable one.

§__121 [Reserved]

§__.122 Use of Federal funds.

Federal funds administered by a department or agency may not be expended for research involving human subjects unless the requirements of this policy have been satisfied.

§__.123 Early termination of research support; evaluation of applications and proposals.

(a) The department or agency head may require that department or agency support for any project be terminated or suspended in the manner prescribed in applicable program requirements, when the department or agency head finds an institution has materially failed to comply with the terms of this policy.

(b) In making decisions about supporting or approving applications or proposals covered by this policy the department or agency head may take into account, in addition to all other eligibility requirements and program criteria, factors such as whether the applicant has been subject to a termination or suspension under paragraph (a) of this section and whether the applicant or the person or persons who would direct or has have directed the scientific and technical aspects of an activity has have, in the judgment of the department or agency head, materially failed to discharge responsibility for the protection of the rights and welfare of human subjects (whether or not the research was subject to federal regulation).

§__.124 Conditions.

With respect to any research project or any class of research projects the department or agency head may impose additional conditions prior to or at the time of approval when in the judgment of the department or agency head additional conditions are necessary for the protection of human subjects.

Abbreviations

AAHRPP. Association for the Accreditation of Human Research Protection Programs
AAU. Association of American Universities
ACRP. Association for Clinical Research Professionals
ADR. adverse drug reaction
AE. adverse event
AMA. American Medical Association
ARENA. Applied Research Ethics National Association

Belmont. *The Belmont Report,* Report of the National Commission for the Protection of Human Subjects of Biomedical and Behavioral Research, reprinted in Appendix C

CFR. *Code of Federal Regulations*
CFO. chief financial officer
CIM. certified IRB manager: accreditation awarded by NAIM
CIOMS. Council for International Organizations of Medical Sciences
CIP. certified IRB professional: accreditation awarded by ARENA
CIRB. central institutional review board
CME. continuing medical education
COC. certificate of confidentiality
COI. conflict of interest
"Common Rule," The. 45 *CFR* 4, reprinted in Appendix D
CRA. clinical research associate
CRB. central review board
CRF. case report form
CRO. contract/clinical research organization
CRC. clinical research coordinator

DEA. U.S. Drug Enforcement Agency
Declaration of Helsinki. Written by the World Medical Association, reprinted in Appendix B
DHEW. U.S. Department of Health, Education and Welfare
DHHS. U.S. Department of Health and Human Services
DIA. Drug Information Association
DOE. U.S. Department of Energy
DSMB. data safety monitoring board

ECG. electrocardiogram
EIR. establishment inspection report

FDA. U.S. Food and Drug Administration
FOIA. Freedom of Information Act
FWA. federalwide assurance

GAO. General Accounting Office
GCP. good clinical practice
GPG. Good Clinical Practice Guidelines

Helsinki. See *Declaration of Helsinki*
HIPAA. Health Insurance Portability and Accountability Act
HPA. human protections administrator
HRP. human research protections
HSR. health services research
HUD. humanitarian use device

IB. investigator's brochure
IBC. institutional biosafety committee
IC. informed consent
ICD. informed consent document
ICF. informed consent form
ICH. International Conference on Harmonisation of Technical Requirements for Registration of Pharmaceuticals for Human Use
ICMJE. International Committee of Medical Journal Editors
IDE. investigational device exemption
IEC. independent/institutional ethics committee
IND. investigational new drug
IO. institutional official
IOM. Institute of Medicine
IRB. institutional review board
IRC. Independent Review Consulting, Inc.

JCAHO. Joint Commission on Accreditation of Healthcare Organizations

MDRS. Medical Device Reporting System
MI. myocardial infarction

NAI. no action indicated
NAIM. National Association of IRB Managers
NBAC. National Bioethics Advisory Commission
NCI. National Cancer Institute
NCPHSBBR. National Commission for the Protection of Human Subjects of Biomedical and Behavioral Research
NCQA. National Committee for Quality Assurance
NDA. new drug application
NHRPAC. National Human Research Protections Advisory Committee
NIH. National Institutes of Health
NOHRPO. National Office of Human Research Protection Oversight
NSF. National Science Foundation
Nuremberg Code, The—"Permissible Medical Experiments," *Trials of War Criminals before the Nuernberg Military Tribunals,* reprinted in Appendix A

OAI. official action indicated
OGCP. Office for Good Clinical Practice
OHRP. Office of Human Research Protections (formerly OPRR)
OIG. Office of the Inspector General
OPRR. Office for Protection from Research Risks
ORA. Office of Regulatory Affairs
ORI. Office of Research Integrity
OSHA. U.S. Occupational Safety and Health Administration

PHRP. Partnership for Human Research Protection
PHS. U.S. Public Health Service
PhRMA. Pharmaceutical Manufacturers of America
PHI. protected health information
PI. principal investigator
PRIM&R. Public Responsibility in Medicine & Research

QA. quality assurance
QC. quality control
QI. quality improvement

RCR. responsible conduct of research

SAE. serious adverse event
SMO. site management organization
SoCRA. Society of Clinical Research Associates
SOP. standard operating procedure
SQA. Society of Quality Assurance
SRA. Society of Research Administrators

VAI. voluntary action indicated

WHO. World Health Organization
WMA. World Medical Association

Glossary of Lay Terms for Use in Preparing Informed Consent Documents

absorb. Take up fluids, take into the body.
acidosis. Condition when blood contains more acid than normal.
acuity. Clearness, keenness, especially of vision, hearing.
acute. New, recent, sudden.
adenopathy. Swollen lymph nodes.
adjuvant. Helpful, assisting, aiding.
adjuvant treatment. Added treatment.
adverse effect. Side-effect of a drug that is undesirable; examples include discomfort or harm to an organ or tissue.
allergic reaction. May include rash, trouble breathing, fever, and/or diarrhea.
ambulate/-ation/-ory. Walk, able to walk.
anaphylaxis. Serious, potentially life-threatening allergic reaction including reduced blood pressure and difficulty breathing.
anemia. Decreased red blood cells; low red blood cell count which can cause tiredness or fatigue
anesthetic (general). A drug or agent used to produce unconsciousness and to decrease the feeling of pain; it puts you to sleep to allow surgery.
anesthetic (local). A drug or agent used to numb an area of your body to permit surgery or biopsy.
angina. Chest pain from too little blood flow to the heart.
angina pectoris. Chest pain from too little blood flow to the heart.
antecubital. Area inside the elbow.
antibiotic. Drug that kills bacteria and other germs.
antibody. Protein made in the body in response to a foreign substance; attacks the foreign substance and protects you from infection.
anticonvulsant. Drug used to prevent or treat seizures.
antilipidemic. A drug that decreases the level of fat(s) in the blood.
antimicrobial. Drug that kills bacteria and other germs.
antiretroviral. Drug used to treat HIV or other diseases caused by viruses.
antiviral. Drug used to treat diseases caused by viruses.
antitussive. A drug used to reduce coughing.
arrhythmia. Any change from the normal heartbeat (abnormal heartbeat).
aspiration. Material entering the lungs following vomiting.
assay. Lab test.
assess. To learn about.
asthma. A lung disease associated with narrowing of the breathing passages in the lungs.
asymptomatic. Without symptoms.
axilla. Armpit.
benign. Not harmful, usually without serious consequences, but with some exceptions, for example, a benign brain tumor may have serious consequences.

b.i.d. Twice a day.
binding/bound. Carried by/stuck together/transported.
bioavailability. The portion of a drug that enters the blood; relates to drugs taken by mouth.
blood profile. Series of blood tests.
bolus. An amount given all at once.
bone mass/density. The amount of calcium in a given amount of bone.
bradyarrhythmias. Slow, irregular heartbeats
bradycardi. Slow heartbeat.
bronchoalveolar lavage. Wash out part of the lung with salt water to obtain lung cells for laboratory tests.
bronchoscopy. Insertion of a flexible tube through the nose and voice box to examine the inside of the lung.
bronchospasm. Narrowing of the breathing passages of the lung causing difficulty breathing and wheezing.
carcinogenic. Capable of causing cancer.
carcinoma. Type of cancer.
cardiac. Refers to the heart.
cardioversion. Return of the normal heartbeat by electric shock or drugs.
catheter. A tube inserted into the body for withdrawing or introducing fluids (for example, a Foley catheter).
catheter (indwelling epidural). A tube placed near the nerves in the spinal cord used to administer anesthesia during an operation.
cerebral trauma. Damage to the brain.
congestive heart disease. Hardening of the arteries of the heart.
chemotherapy. Treatment of disease, usually cancer, by drugs.
chronic. Continuing for a long time.
clinical. Referring to medical care.
clinical trial. An experiment involving patients.
cognitive tests. Tests of thinking abilities.
complete response. Total disappearance of disease.
consolidation phase. Treatment phase intended to make a remission permanent follows induction.
contraindicated. Should not be used.
control. Healthy volunteer.
controlled trial. Study in which the experimental treatment or procedure is compared to a standard (control) treatment or procedure.
cooperative group. Association of multiple hospitals and doctors to perform clinical trials together.
coronary. Refers to the blood vessels that supply the heart.
coronary heart disease. Hardening of the arteries of the heart.
CT scan (CAT) (computerized tomography). Computerized series of x-rays.
culture. Test for infection or germs that could cause infection.
CVA (cerebrovascular accident). Stroke.
diastolic. Lower number in blood pressure reading.
distal. Toward the end, away from the center of the body.
diuretic. A water pill or drug that causes an increase in urination.
doppler. Sound waves.
double blind. Study in which neither investigators nor subjects know what drug the subject is receiving.
dysplasia. Abnormal cells.
echocardiogram. Sound wave test of the heart.
edema. Increased fluid in body tissues, swelling.
EEG (electroencephalogram). Recording of the electric waves in the brain.
efficacy. Effectiveness; how well something works.
electrocardiogram. ECG or EKG, electrical tracing of the heart.
electrolyte imbalance. Imbalance of minerals in the blood (for example, potassium or sodium).
emesis. Vomiting.
empiric. Based on experience.
endoscopic. Insertion of a flexible tube with

a light to examine an internal part of the body.

enteral. Given through the stomach or intestines.

epidemiologic. Referring to the study or the distribution and populations of characteristics and diseases.

epidural. A tube placed near the nerves in the spinal cord to administer anesthesia during operation.

extravasate. To leak outside of a blood vessel.

FDA. U.S. Food and Drug Administration, the branch of the federal government that approves new drugs.

fibrillation. Irregular beat of the heart or other muscle.

gastrointestinal. Relating to the stomach and intestines.

general anesthesia. A drug or agent used to produce unconsciousness and to decrease the feeling of pain; it puts you to sleep to allow surgery.

glucose. A sugar.

gout. A disease that causes a painful inflammation of the joints.

hematocrit. Amount of red blood cells in the blood.

hematoma. A bruise; a black and blue mark.

hemodynamic measuring. Measuring of blood flow.

hemoglobin. A substance in the blood that carries oxygen.

hemolysis. Breakdown of red blood cells.

heparin lock. A plastic tube filled with blood thinner that is placed in a vein to give injections or take out blood.

hepatic. Refers to the liver.

hepatoma. Cancer or tumor of the liver.

holter monitor. A portable machine for recording heartbeats over a period of time.

hypercalcemia. Increased level of calcium in the blood.

hyperkalemia. Increased level of potassium in the blood.

hypernatremia. Increased level of sodium in the blood.

hypertension. High blood pressure.

hypocalcemia. Reduced level of calcium in the blood.

hyponatremia. Reduced level of sodium in the blood.

hypotension. Low blood pressure.

hypoxemia. A decrease of oxygen in the blood.

hypoxia. A decrease of oxygen in the blood.

iatrogenic. Injury caused by a physician or by treatment.

IDE. Investigational device exemption; the license to test an unapproved new medical device.

idiopathic. A disorder for which the cause is unknown.

illicit drugs/substances. Illegal drugs.

immune system. The system in the body that reacts to foreign or occasionally one's own proteins.

immunoglobulin. A substance produced by the body that binds to a foreign substance

immunosuppressive. Drug which reduces the body's immune response, used in transplantation and diseases caused by disordered immunity.

immunotherapy. Use of drugs to help the body's immune (protective) system; usually used to destroy cancer cells.

IND. Investigational new drug; the license to test an unapproved new drug.

induction phase. Beginning phase or stage of a treatment.

induration. Hardening.

infarct. Death of tissue because of lack of blood supply.

infusion. Introduction of a substance into the body, usually into the blood through a vein

ingestion. Eating; taking by mouth.

intramuscular. Into the muscle; within the muscle

intrathecal. Injected into the space around the spinal cord.

intravenous (IV). Injected into a vein.

intravesical. In the bladder.
intubation (tracheal). The placement of a tube into the throat (trachea) to assist breathing.
invasive procedure. Puncture, opening, or cutting of the skin.
ischemia. Decreased oxygen in a tissue (usually because of decreased blood flow).
leukopenia. Low white blood cell count, which can increase the possibility of infection.
lipid content. Fat content in the blood.
local anesthesia. A drug or agent used to numb an area of your body to permit surgery or biopsy.
localized. Restricted to one area, limited to one area.
lumen. The cavity of an organ or tube (for example, a blood vessel).
lymphangiography. An x-ray of the lymph nodes or tissues after injection of dye in lymph vessels (for example, in feet).
lymphocyte. A type of white blood cell important in immunity and defense against infection.
lymphoma. A cancer of the lymph nodes (or tissues).
lumbar puncture. Spinal tap; placement of a needle between the bones in the back to remove some of the fluid around the spinal cord.
malaise. A vague feeling of bodily discomfort, feeling bad.
malignancy. Cancer or other progressively enlarging and spreading tumor, usually fatal if not successfully treated.
medulloblastoma. A type of brain tumor.
megaloblastosis. Change in red blood cells.
metabolize. Process of breaking down substances in cells to obtain energy.
metastasis. Spread of cancer cells from one part of the body to another.
MI (myocardial infarction). Heart attack.
minimal. Slight.
minimize. Reduce.
monitor. Check on; keep track of; watch carefully.
mobility. Ease of movement.
morbidity. Undesired result or complication.
mortality. Death or death rate.
MRI. Magnetic resonance imaging; body pictures created using magnetic rather than x-ray energy.
mucosa/mucous membrane. Moist lining of digestive, respiratory, reproductive and urinary tracts.
myocardial. Referring to the heart.
myocardial infarction. Heart attack.
nasogastric tube. Tube from the nose to the stomach.
NCI. National Cancer Institute.
necrosis. Death of tissue.
neonatal. Referring to the newborn period.
neoplasia. Tumor, may be benign or malignant.
neuroblastoma. A cancer of the nerve tissue.
neutropenia. Decrease in the main part of the white blood cells.
NIH. National Institutes of Health.
noninvasive. Not breaking, cutting, or entering the skin.
normal subject. Healthy volunteer.
nosocomial pneumonia. Pneumonia acquired in the hospital.
occlusion. Closing; obstruction.
oncology. The study of tumors or cancer.
ophthalmic. Referring to the eye.
optimal. Best, most favorable or desirable.
oral administration. By mouth.
orthopedic. Referring to the bones.
osteopetrosis. Rare bone disorder characterized dense bone.
osteoporosis. Softening of the bones.
ovaries. Female sex glands.
parenteral. Injection of a drug into a vein or into the skin.
patency. Condition of being open.
pathogenesis. Causative mechanism in disease.

percutaneous. Through the skin.
perforation. A tear or a hole.
perinatal. Referring to the pregnancy and newborn period.
per os (PO). By mouth.
pharmacokinetics. The study of the way the body absorbs, distributes, metabolizes, and gets rid of a drug.
phase I. Initial study of a new drug in humans to determine the limits of tolerance and its safety.
phase II. Second phase of a study of a new drug intended to obtain initial information.
phase III. Large scale trials to confirm and expand information on safety and usefulness of a new drug.
phlebitis. Irritation or inflammation of the vein.
placebo. A substance with no active medication.
placebo effect. The perception of improvement when a placebo is given.
platelets. Small particles in the blood that help with clotting.
postoperative. After surgery.
potentiate. Increase or multiply the effect of a drug or toxin by administration of another drug or toxin at the same time.
potentiator. An agent that helps another agent work well.
preoperative. Before surgery.
PRN. As needed.
prophylaxis. A drug given to prevent disease or infection.
prognosis. Chances for recovery.
progresses. Worsens, gets worse.
prone. Lying on the stomach.
prospective. Study following patients forward in time.
protocol. Plan of study.
proximal. Closer to the center of the body, away from the end.
pulmonary. Referring to the lungs.
q.d. Everyday.
radiation therapy. X-ray or cobalt treatment.
random. By chance.
randomization. Chance selection, like flipping a coin.
RBC. Red blood cell.
recombinant. Formation of new combinations of genes resulting from the manipulation of genes in the laboratory.
reconstitution. Putting back together the original parts or elements; for drugs; preparation of a drug for administration by adding liquid to a dry, powdered drug.
refractory. Not responding to treatment.
regeneration. Regrowth of a structure or of lost tissue.
relapse. The return of a disease.
remission. Disappearance of evidence of cancer or other disease.
renal. Referring to the kidneys.
replicable. Possible to duplicate.
resect. Remove or cut out surgically.
resolve. Go away.
retrospective study. Study looking back over past experience.
sedation. Giving medicine to make someone sleepy or less anxious.
seizures. Intense uncontrollable movements.
sequelae. A condition following as a consequence of a disease.
sequential. In a row.
serum. Blood.
spirometry/PFT. Measurement of how well you breathe and how well your lungs function.
subcutaneous. Under the skin.
supine. Lying on the back.
systolic. Top number in blood pressure reading.
terminate. Stop.
thoracic. Relating to the chest.
thrombocytopenia. A condition in which there is an abnormally small amount of platelets in the blood.
thrombosis. Blood clot.

toxicity. An unwanted side-effect resulting in injury to a tissue or organ.
toxicology test. A test for illegal drugs.
tracheal intubation. The placement of a tube into the throat (trachea) to assist breathing.
transient. Lasting or staying only a short time
venipuncture. Blood drawing.
vertigo. Dizziness.

Useful Websites

ORGANIZATIONS

Agency for Healthcare Policy and Research (AHCPR). *www.ahcpr.gov*

Archives of the National Human Research Protections Advisory Committee (NHRPAC). *http://ohrp.osophs.dhhs.gov/nhrpac/nhrpac.htm*

Association for Clinical Research Professionals (ACRP). *www.acrpnet.org*

The Belmont Report. *http://ohrp.osophs.dhhs.gov/humansubjects/guidance/belmont.htm*

CenterWatch. An information source for the clinical trials industry, *www.centerwatch.com*

Code of Federal Regulations (CFR). *http://www.access.gpo.gov/nara/cfr/*

Department of Health and Human Services (DHHS) Office of the Inspector General (OIG). *http://oig.hhs.gov*

Drug Information Association (DIA). *http://www.diahome.org/docs/index.cfm*

Expedited Review Categories, OHRP. See Office for Human Research Protections

Food and Drug Administration (FDA)

Clinical investigators who have provided adequate assurances re: future compliance. *http://www.fda.gov/ora/compliance_ref/bimo/asurlist.htm*

Debarment list. *http://www.fda.gov/ora/compliance_ref/debar/default.htm*

Disqualified list. *http://www.fda.gov/ora/compliance_ref/bimo/disqlist.htm*

Electronic mailing lists. Free lists to keep up to date on the FDA's activities and the products it regulates: *http://www.fda.gov/emaillist.html*

Homepage. *www.FDA.gov*

Information for health professionals. *http://www.fda.gov/oc/oha/default.htm#clinical*

Information sheets. *http://www.fda.gov/oc/ohrt/irbs/default.htm*

Notice of initiation of disqualification proceedings and opportunity to explain. *www.fda.gov/foi/nidpoe/default.html*

Restricted list. *http://www.fda.gov/ora/compliance_ref/bimo/restlist.htm*

Warning letters. *http://www.fda.gov/foi/warning.htm*

Helsinki, Declaration of. See World Medical Association

ICH. See International Conference on Harmonisation

Institute of Medicine (IOM). *http://www.iom.edu/hrrp*

International Conference on Harmonisation (ICH). *http://www.ich.org/*

MedWatch. *http://www.fda.gov/medwatch*

NHRPAC. See Archives of the National Human Research Protections Advisory Committee

National Institutes of Health (NIH).

Bioethics resources. *http://www.nih.gov/sigs/bioethics*

Grants and funding opportunities. *http://grants.nih.gov/grants/index.cfm*

Office of Human Subjects Research. *http://ohsr.od.nih.gov*

President's Council on Bioethics. *http://bioethics.gov*

Office for Civil Rights.

HIPAA. *http://www.hhs.gov/ocr/hipaa/*

Office for Human Research Protections (OHRP).

Common findings and guidance. *http://ohrp.osophs.dhhs.gov/references/findings.pdf*

Expedited review categories. *http://ohrp.osophs.dhhs.gov/humansubjects/guidance/expedited98.htm*

Guidance documents. *http://ohrp.osophs.dhhs.gov/g-topics.htm*

Guidance on written IRB procedures. *http://ohrp.osophs.dhhs.gov/humansubjects/guidance/wirbproc.pdf*

Homepage. *http://ohrp.osophs.dhhs.gov/*

Policy guidance page. *http://ohrp.osophs.dhhs.gov/polasur.htm*

Office of Human Subjects Research. See National Institutes of Health, Office of Human Subjects Research

Office of Research Integrity. *http://ori.dhhs.gov/*

Public Health Service.

Administrative actions. *http://silk.nih.gov/public/cbz1bje.@www.orilist.html*

Public Responsibility in Medicine & Research (PRIM&R). *http://www.primr.org*

World Medicial Association (WMA). Author of *World Medical Association Declaration of Helsinki. http://www.wma.net/e/home.html*

POPULAR LISTSERVS

The Office for Human Research Protections (OHRP).

The Office for Human Research Protections (OHRP) created a LISTSERV to provide interested individuals with information regarding human subject research protection, upcoming educational workshops, and other programs. The list is used for posting human subject research protection announcements only; it is not a discussion list. You may post an announcement for an upcoming workshop or conference, and the editor will review/OK it for inclusion.

Subscribe to the OHRP-L LISTSERV by sending an e-mail to *listserv@ list.nih.gov with* the following text in the message body:

SUBSCRIBE OHRP-L Firstname Lastname [Replace Firstname and Lastname with your name].

LISTSERV will get your e-mail address from the "From:" address of your e-mail message.

If at any time you wish to unsubscribe from the list, send an e-mail to *listserv@list.nih.gov* with the following text in the message body:

UNSUBSCRIBE OHRP-L

For additional information about NIH LISTSERV visit *http://list.nih.gov/.*

The IRB Forum.
www.IRBForum.org
(formerly www. McWIRB.org)

The IRB Forum (previously known as "MCWIRB") promotes the discussion of ethical, regulatory, and policy concerns with human subjects research. The IRB Forum strives to create an atmosphere for open and respectful conversation about issues of mutual interest to the members. Although the privacy of e-mail cannot be guaranteed, the members of The IRB Forum should respect the confidentiality and opinions of others on the list. Please review the features, policy, and procedures of The IRB Forum before requesting membership. Individuals who fail to abide by the terms of membership are subject to removal from The IRB Forum.

The IRB Forum is open to past and current members of institutional review boards (IRBs) or research ethics committees (REC), IRB/REC administrators, individuals involved in IRB/REC oversight, and others with professional involvement in IRB/REC and/or research activities. Others will be admitted if their involvement in human subjects research will contribute to the discussion of issues pertinent to The IRB Forum. International participants are welcome. There is no membership fee.

List of Sample Forms

Figures

List of Contributors

EDITORS

Deirdre Hall, CCRC, CCRA, CIP, is Manager for Quality Standards at Pfizer Pharmaceuticals Group, New York, N.Y.

Eileen Hilton, MD, is President and CEO of the Biomedical Research Alliance of New York, Great Neck, N.Y., and is a Professor of Clinical Medicine at Albert Einstein College of Medicine.

CONTRIBUTING WRITERS

Kendra Dimond, Esq., is a Partner at the National Health Law Practice of Epstein Becker & Green, P.C., Washington, D.C.

Raffaella Hart, CIP, is Director of the IRB at the Biomedical Research Alliance of New York, Great Neck, N.Y.

Kimberly Irvine, BS, is Vice President of Operations at the Biomedical Research Alliance of New York, Great Neck, N.Y.

Mary R. Marta, Esq., is an Associate at the National Health Law Practice of Epstein Becker & Green, P.C., Washington, D.C.

Philip D. Mitchell, Esq., is a Partner at the National Health Law Practice of Epstein Becker & Green, P.C., New York, N.Y., and Newark, N.J.

Elaine V. Neal, CIP, is Assistant Director of the Office of the IRB at the North Shore-Long Island Jewish Health System, Lake Success, N.Y.

Lillian Oshva, MD, is an Attending Physician in the Emergency Department of the New York University School of Medicine; and is a Member of the IRB at the Biomedical Research Alliance of New York, Great Neck, N.Y.

Linda Reuter, MS, CIP, is a Policy Specialist in the North Shore-Long Island Jewish Health System, Office of the IRB, Lake Success, N.Y.

Kay Ryan, CIP, New York University School of Medicine, New York, N.Y.

Victor W. Sidel, MD, is a Distinguished University Professor of Social Medicine at Montefiore Medical Center and Albert Einstein College of Medicine, Adjunct Professor of Public Health at Weill Medical College of Cornell University, Chair of the IRB at Montefiore Medical Center, and Chair of the IRB at the Biomedical Research Alliance of New York, Great Neck, N.Y.

EDITORIAL BOARD

Ruth G. Abramson, MD, now deceased, was Associate Dean for Research at Mount Sinai School of Medicine, Chairperson of the Mount Sinai School of Medicine IRB, and Professor of Medicine (Nephrology), New York, N.Y., when this book was written.

Jacki Altman is Director of the Office of the IRB and Director of the Office of Grants and Contracts at North Shore-Long Island Jewish Health System, Lake Success, N.Y.

Erica Heath, MBA, CIP, is President of IRC-Independent Review Consulting, San Anselmo, Calif.

Printed in the United States
27815LVS00002B/1-44

9 781555 720834